The
ABCs of
Prostate
Cancer

The Book That
Could Save Your Life

Joseph E. Oesterling, M.D.

Mark A. Moyad, M.P.H.

MADISON BOOKS

Lanham • New York • Oxford

Back cover photos: *top row, left to right:*
Justice Paul Stevens, Marv Levy, Richard Petty and Jerry VerDorn.
Bottom row, left to right: Robert Novak, Bob Watson, Jim Ferree and Michael Milken.

Front cover photos: *top to bottom and left to right:*
Robert Dole, Sidney Poitier, Stan Musial, Jerry Lewis, H. Norman Schwarzkopf,
Len Dawson, Robert Goulet and Mayor Marion Barry.

Editor

Kristen K. Lidke

Wordplay

Design and Production

Judalyn G. Seling

Seling Design

Illustrator

Marlene W. DenHouter

BMC Media Services

University of Michigan Medical Center

Printer

Edwards Brothers Inc.

Ann Arbor, Mich.

Published by Madison Books
4720 Boston Way
Lanham, Maryland 20706

12 Hid's Copse Road
Cummor Hill
Oxford OX2 9JJ, England

Library of Congress Cataloging-in-Publication Data

Oesterling, Joseph E.
    The ABCs of prostate cancer : the book that could save your life /
Joseph E. Oesterling, Mark A. Moyad.
        p.   cm.
    Includes index.
    ISBN 1–56833–085–5 (cloth : alk. paper)
    1. Prostate—Cancer—Popular works. I. Moyad, Mark A., 1965–
II. Title.
RC280.P7037 1997
616.99'463—dc21   *96–48316*
                                                              CIP

ISBN 1–56833–085–5 (cloth : alk. paper)
ISBN 1–56833–097–9 (pbk : alk. paper)

Distributed by National Book Network

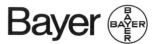

Pharmaceutical Division

Jo Ellen Schweinle, MD
Director
Scientific Relations

Dear Doctor:

We at Bayer Corporation, Pharmaceutical Division, maker of Cipro® I.V. (ciprofloxacin) and Cipro® (ciprofloxacin HCl) Tablets, are pleased to present you with *The ABC's of Prostate Cancer: The Book That Could Save Your Life*, a user-friendly guide about prostate cancer for patients and their families.

Written in a manner that is appropriate for individuals with either limited <u>or</u> extensive knowledge about the disease, the book addresses the more frequently asked and important questions about prostate cancer.

We trust that this reference guide will be a valuable tool in helping you to educate patients and their families about prostate cancer and its treatment.

Cordially,

Schweinle, M.D.

Jo Ellen Schweinle, MD
Director, Scientific Relations

Bayer Corporation
400 Morgan Lane
West Haven, CT 06516-4175

Phone 203 812-6592
Fax 203 812-6547

Dedications

To all of the individuals who contributed to this book. Without their commitment, it could never have been possible. Thank you!

To our family members (and everyone else) who have battled or are battling with cancer today. We are going to find a cure for this thing one day soon!

— Joseph E. Oesterling and Mark A. Moyad

To my wonderful wife, Carmen. Nothing in my career could have been possible without her endless sacrifice and total support. She is my best friend, and I will love her always!

To my children, Christopher and Jennifer, who always greet Daddy at the door with unconditional love and wholehearted enthusiasm even though Daddy has not been around enough.

To my father, Walter, who died of prostate cancer. To me, he was the most brilliant and humble man in the world. Every day I refer to one of his "pearls of wisdom."

To my mother, Leona, who taught me discipline, commitment to excellence, and dedication to hard work — virtues that I will carry with me my whole life.

To my sister, Janet, as humble as my father and as dedicated as my mother. She is always there for me. I will continually remember her early morning telephone calls.

To my older brother, Robert, my adviser and the person who motivated me to attend college. Without his encouragement, I would not be a physician today.

To my younger brother, Mark, who has been and will always be one of my closest friends. I will never forget our early days playing and working together on the family farm.

— Joseph E. Oesterling

To my father, Dr. Robert H. Moyad, who is not just a great physician but, more important, a great father and the No. 1 role model in my life.

To my mother, Eva, my best friend and someone whose contributions to my life have been and continue to be immeasurable.

To my older brother, Andrew, who has always been there for me during the rain and the sunshine, and who has dedicated his life to making this world a better place.

To my younger brother, Tom, an individual with unlimited potential and who as a doctor will be one of the best around.

Last, but never least, Dr. Joseph E. Oesterling, a person I hope to have the pleasure of working with the rest of my life.

— Mark A. Moyad

Special Acknowledgments

To M. Brooke Moran and all the people at the American Foundation for Urologic Disease (AFUD) and the American Urological Association (AUA) — thank you for your continued commitment to the cause.

– Joseph E. Oesterling and Mark A. Moyad

To my superb assistant, Marilyn Smith. I have never worked with a more compassionate, sincere and dedicated individual. She is *always* there, ready to contribute, whether it is 6 a.m. or 11 p.m., Monday or Saturday. Indeed, as Mark Moyad would say, "Marilyn Smith is a gift from God."

To Dr. Patrick C. Walsh, always my mentor and father in the field of urology. He is one of the most brilliant and skillful urologic surgeons in the world.

– Joseph E. Oesterling

To Dr. Anvita Sinha, a dedicated and compassionate physician who over the years provided me with advice and support.

To Julie Savalas, one of the most inspirational individuals I have ever met and a true lifelong friend.

– Mark A. Moyad

Acknowledgements

A

Dr. and Mrs. Bernard Agranoff
Will Agranoff
Dr. Muzammil Ahmed
Dr. Faxil Tuncay Aki
Dr. Ameena Al-dabbagh
Abdullah Nussein Al-dabbagh
American Cancer Society
Lars Andersson
Pat Anthony
Dr. Sami Arap
Dr. Gary Arendash
Dr. Hussein Awang

B

Rick Bachrach
Karin Bahrs
Raymone Bain
Dr. Manuel Bayona
Dr. Mario Bcduschi
Tex Beha
Dr. William D. Belville
Scott A. Berchtold
Alex Berry
Dr. Paul Bessette
Jim Blow
Dr. David A. Bloom
Martha Jane Bonkemeyer
Dr. Ola Bratt
Dr. Robert L. Bree
Dr. Stuart Brooks
Dr. Rita Bruce
Mary Buckley
Deborah Burch
Dr. Wayne Burnette
William J. Busse

C

Dr. Richard Campo
Dr. Ted Chang
Jack Cichon
Prissi Cohen
Randy & Heidi Colucci
Kathleen Connoley
Dr. Kathleen Cooney

Donald Costley
Don Coucke
Kaerensa Craft
Debra Crumby

D

Susan D'Agostini
Daniel Designer Photography Inc.
Janice Davis
Dr. Mark Day
Dr. Ann DeBaldo
Jacques Demichelis
Jane Dickerson
Dr. Stephen Doggett

E

Dr. Barry England

F

Dr. Gary Faerber
Dr. Richard Figge
Lesley M. Finney
Dr. Peter Fischer
Ann Fogleman
Dr. Mark Frydenberg

G

Susan Garrison
Toni Gentilli
Dr. Peter J. Gilling
Lin Goings, photographer
Dr. Keow Mei Goh
Dr. J. Gottesman
Vera Goulet
Dr. Peter Grimm

H

Meg Habenicht
Tom Harbor
Dr. John Harris
Paige Harris
Vicki Hart
Mike and Chrissi Hatfield
Frank Hedge
Dr. Skip Holden

I

Iwamoto Japanese Studio

J

Vera Jackson
Thawin Jariya-Kovit
Missy Jenkins
Andrew Johnson
Norm Johnson
Robert Jors

K

Dr. Michael Kern
Dr. Stephanie J. Kielb
Dr. Eduardo Kleer
Pam Knies
Dr. John W. Konnak
Dr. Harry Koo
Ginny Koops
Dr. Tomohiko Koyanagi
Dr. David Kraklau
Bonnie Krauss
Wendy Kruzel
Dr. Boo Kwa

L

Linda Lacey and all of the parents,
    students and teachers at Lee
    Academy (Tampa, Fla.)
Cathy Lash
Dr. Jon K. Lattimer
Lynn Leach
Dr. Paul Leaverton
Dr. Cheryl Lee
Dr. Young-Goo Lee
Dr. Marcia Lichty
Dr. Ossi Lindell
John-Olof Lofberg
Lawrence V. Lohnhi
Peter and Elisa Losee
Susan Lovett
George Lowe

M

Dr. Jill Macoska
Dr. Aziz Fam Mankarious
Dr. Robert Marcovich
A.P. Marshall

Andrew Manning
Dr. T.P. Mate
Eric McClenaghan
Mylinda McCoy
Don McGinnis
Dr. David G. McLeod
Dr. James E. Montie
Marilyn Mulla
Dr. Stephanie Myers

N

Sankar A. Nair
Dr. Roberta Nespoli
Non Surgical Prostate
    Cancer Center
Northwest Tumor Institute

O

Kimberly A. O'Brien
Dr. Dana Alan Ohl
Dr. Ann Olendorf
Bob Olson
Dr. Haluk Ozen

P

Dr. Dalibor Pacik
Dr. Kenneth Palmer
Jerry Pam
Dr. Ravat Panvichian
Dr. John Park
Barbara Payne & Payne
    Communications
Diane Pawlecki
Dr. Lester Persky
Dorothy L. Petersen
John and Karen Peterson
Dr. Doris Phillips
Dr. Kenneth Pienta
Nellie A. Pitts
Robert & Colleen Piscetta

Dr. Armando Plata
Dr. Edson Pontes
Pamela Poitier
Dr. Dmitri Yu Pushkar

R

Katie Ralston
Jim and Tammy Ramirez
Bette Rank
Dr. Michael G. Rashid
Michael Reese
Lisa F. Rhodes
Dr. Thomas Richardson
Dr. Jose Arturo Rodriguez Rivera
Sr. Miguel Navarro Robledo
John Robus
Doug Rogers
Jim Rosbolt
Dr. Joan Rose
Dr. Partha Roy
Dr. Sandip Roy
Ed Runser
Phil Rupp

S

Dr. Wael Sakr
Dr. Martin G. Sanda
Jose Pedro dos Santos
Dr. Fazul Sarkar
Dr. Alvaro S. Sarkis
Sheldon Schwartz
Dr. Brian D. Seifman
Ann Marie Septer
Julia Simmons
Paul Slater
Ronald Snead
Dean Robert Sokol, M.D.
Joe Stabile
Dawn Street
Steves Photography Inc.
Swedish Medical Center
    Tumor Institute

T

Bill Tate
Dr. Marie-Blanche Tchetgen
Dr. Anita Tekchandani
Dr. Serdar Tekgul
Paul Thacker, photographer
Dr. Alberto Trinchieri
Dr. Kjell Tueter

U

Johnny Unitas Jr.

V

Dr. Christopher Vallorosi
Dr. Carl VanAppledorn
Dr. Apoorva Vashi
Shawn Vass
Dr. Ann Vickery

W

Martha Ward
William Wayman
Gary Wedemeyer
Peri Weingrad
Bruce Weintraub
Joseph A. Welch, photographer
Maria White
Susan E. Whitlam
Dr. James Williams
Dr. Jeffrey F. Williams
Lynn Williams
Dr. Manfred Wirth
Jeff Witjas
Dr. Kirk Wojno
Dr. Stuart Wolf

Z

Dr. Marc Zerbib

Our Team

We'd like to thank the members of our team who helped shape our thoughts and words into the book you're now reading:

Editor Kristen K. Lidke, owner of Wordplay, an Ann Arbor-based editing service, and former science writer for the University of Michigan Medical Center. For more than 10 years she served as managing editor of *Advance*, the magazine of the U-M Hospitals, Medical School and School of Nursing. Lidke has won more than two dozen national, regional and statewide awards for medical feature writing and publication excellence.

Designer and production coordinator Judalyn G. Seling, owner of Seling Design of Dexter, Mich., and former senior art director for the University of Michigan Medical Center, Office of Planning and Marketing. A founding member of the American Advertising Federation Ad Club in Ann Arbor, Seling has won more than two dozen national, regional and statewide awards for design excellence.

Illustrator Marlene W. DenHouter, a staff illustrator at the University of Michigan Medical School whose work has appeared in numerous medical journals and books. She holds a master of fine arts degree in medical and biological illustration from the University of Michigan.

Contents

Preface

It was July 1987, and the summer hay-bailing season was in full swing at the Oesterling farm in south central Indiana. Everyone was working hard and feeling well. At the time my father, Walter, was 75 years old, feeling better than ever and more health-conscious than anyone I knew. He ate a low-fat, high-fiber diet, avoided desserts, exercised regularly to maintain muscle tone and a handsome physique, and he got eight hours of sleep every night so he would awake in the morning feeling rested. However, he neglected one very important thing: to have his prostate examined annually.

Little did anyone realize that hot summer day that my father had incurable prostate cancer that would take his life in less than four years.

While loading the hay wagons with him on the afternoon of July 7, I convinced him to come back with me to The Johns Hopkins Hospital in Baltimore, Md., for a prostate checkup. At that time, I was a urology resident-in-training there under the mentorship of Patrick C. Walsh, M.D. When my father saw Dr. Walsh three days later, he was found to have a rock-hard prostate gland upon digital-rectal examination. A prostate biopsy confirmed the presence of cancer. Three weeks later, he underwent lymph-node biopsy and prostate-removal surgery. Two of his lymph nodes contained cancer, indicating that the disease was incurable, as it had already spread outside of the prostate gland.

In the years that followed, my devoted mother, Leona, and the rest of the family struggled with my father's illness. After he was diagnosed, not a day went by that my father didn't worry. Living under the shadow of cancer, he said, was like being trapped inside a cage with a baby lion. In the beginning, the lion was small and unthreatening, but he knew that eventually the lion would grow and eventually devour him. Three years after diagnosis, the bone pain began. Then the difficulty urinating. Eventually, the cancer

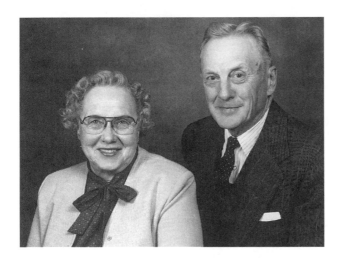

Walter Oesterling, who died of prostate cancer in 1991, and his wife, Leona.

encroached on his spine and my father became paralyzed and bedridden for the last five months of his life. Through it all, my mother, a strong individual, cared for him at home, never complaining, always beside him.

There is no doubt that prostate cancer is a family disease; it is not just a man's problem.

On Jan. 12, 1991, my father, Walter Bernard Oesterling, died of prostate cancer at the age of 79. He succumbed to the disease because he didn't know about the importance of getting an annual prostate exam. He didn't know that the only way to prevent death from prostate cancer is to catch it while it is still at an early, curable — and usually symptomless — stage.

This information could have saved my father's life, as well as the lives of 41,000 men who die annually in the United States from prostate cancer, the most common malignancy in men today.

The inspiration for this book comes from my father's death and my desire to help prevent other such deaths by educating men and their loved ones about the prostate gland, prostate cancer and its treatments.

When I left the Mayo Clinic in Rochester, Minn., in June 1994 to come to the University of Michigan in Ann Arbor, I met Mark Moyad, M.P.H., an expert on world health issues and a respected public educator. He and I spent many hours discussing prostate cancer and ways to prevent men from dying of it. We soon realized that the answer could only come from educating the public.

But first we had to document the need for such education, so we surveyed several hundred men from all walks of life to measure their knowledge about the prostate gland and its disorders. What we found was startling. For example, 42 percent of those surveyed thought that women also have a prostate gland, when in fact the prostate is a male organ. Most thought that prostate cancer could not be inherited when, in reality, it is a familial disease that can be passed on from the mother's or father's side of the family. Indeed, we found a serious need for public education about the prostate and its disorders.

The next step was to determine the most effective method of informing men and their loved ones about prostate cancer. Should it be in the form of an audiotape? A videotape? A short brochure? An in-depth book? Again, a survey told us that most people would prefer a comprehensive yet easy-to-understand book that could be taken anywhere. They also wanted the material to be relatively brief so that it could be read in two to three days. They also wanted the information to be presented in a concise, friendly manner so that it could be remembered easily and located quickly. Little amenities, such as larger print size and extra space to take notes, were also requested.

We also discovered that men wanted to know how the prostate works and where it's located. And while they were most interested in prostate cancer, they also wanted to know how to distinguish this disease from other common disorders of the gland, such as benign prostatic hyperplasia, or BPH (noncancerous enlargement of the prostate). They also wanted to know how prostate cancer is treated, and they expected the various treatment options to be presented in an objective and unbiased manner. Respondents to our survey also sought the latest information about coping with the side effects of treatment, such as incontinence and impotence. In general, they wanted to be informed so that they could work with their physician to determine the best way of managing their disease.

We also learned that men were eager to hear from others who've been treated for prostate cancer. Knowing how to get in touch with local, regional and national support groups was another priority.

Mr. Moyad and I listened to these men and their families' needs and responded by creating the book you are about to read: *The ABCs of Prostate Cancer: The Book That Could Save Your Life.* Its dozen chapters each are organized into three sections labeled A, B and C — hence the name of the book.

In addition to being informative, we hope this book will provide hope and encouragement to those with and without prostate cancer. It includes anecdotes and advice from more than 50 survivors, including those in the spotlight, such as Sen. Robert Dole, Mayor Marion Barry, Gen. H. Norman Schwarzkopf, Jerry Lewis, Robert Goulet, Stan Musial and Len Dawson. Prostate-cancer patients from around the world (including Australia, Greece, Hawaii, Japan, Norway, Russia and Spain) also tell of their encounters with the disease. The testimonies of these survivors are a vital reminder that prostate cancer need not be a death sentence; that men who have the disease, if treated early, can not only survive, but thrive. Finally, you will also hear from those whose voices have been all but ignored during this epidemic: the women. Despite popular thinking, prostate cancer is also a woman's disease.

The message of this book is simple: The prostate gland is important. Take care of it. Get it checked annually. If cancer is found, do not despair; effective, safe treatments are available.

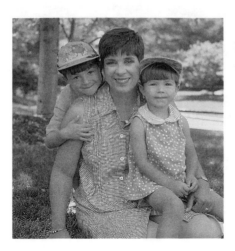

Carmen Oesterling with son Christopher and daughter Jennifer.

With my strong family history of prostate cancer (in addition to my father, my grandfather and a cousin have had it) and the fact that I recently turned 40, I have started getting my own prostate checked each year. It is the least I can do for my wife, Carmen, and our two children, Christopher and Jennifer.

Joseph E. Oesterling, M.D.

July 5, 1996
Ann Arbor, Mich.

Introduction

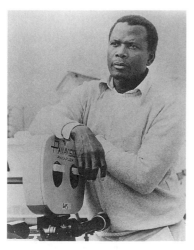

Sidney Poitier

You'll hear a lot of men who've been diagnosed with prostate cancer say they never had a symptom, never felt anything. That's because the most common symptom is no symptom at all.

If you are African American or have a family history of prostate cancer, you need to begin the digital-rectal exam and the PSA blood test at age 40. These tests could save your life. They may sound uncomfortable and may be even down-right frightening, but dying of prostate cancer is a lot more frightening.

And if you are diagnosed, you probably don't even want to think about the possible side effects of treatment, such as problems with erection. But we're talking about treatment that can save your life. The prostate is not vital for sexual activity. You can have sex without a prostate; you can't have sex if you're dead.

The bottom line is that there's a lot that you can do to fight prostate cancer; reading this book is a step in the right direction. Take care of yourself. Eat healthy. Take charge of your medical health. If you don't understand something, ask questions. If you still don't understand, ask *more* questions. Get a second opinion. Call your doctor. Call the American Cancer Society. Talk to people. Tell your friends to get their checkups.

Early detection is the key to fighting this disease, so do yourself and your loved ones a favor: Get a digital-rectal exam and a PSA blood test — it may save your life.

I know; these simple tests saved mine.

Sidney Poitier

Actor

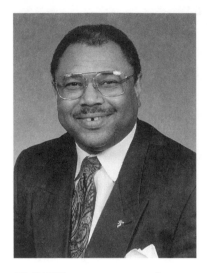

Bob Watson, general manager of the New York Yankees.

In the spring of 1994, after three decades in professional baseball, I was living the life of my dreams. My wife, Carol, and I had recently celebrated our 25th anniversary and, as the first minority to be promoted to general manager of a professional baseball team (the Houston Astros), I was absolutely at the top of my career.

The date for my annual team physical fell on Sunday, April 10, which also happened to be my 47th birthday. But instead of going to the doctor, I elected to spend that fine spring day with my wife. I finally rescheduled the appointment for May, and as part of the exam, I asked the doctor to give me a PSA test in addition to the digital-rectal exam. A couple of scouts I knew had been diagnosed with prostate cancer the year before, and they had urged me to ask for the test.

The doctor said, "No, no, you're too young to do that. We don't start giving the PSA blood test until you're 50 or so; we'll just do the digital-rectal exam."

I insisted. "Nope," I said. "Do the PSA."

Well, the results came back at 5.8, which raised a red flag for our team urologist, who ordered some more tests and a biopsy. Out of the six core biopsies, one came back positive, and it was a particularly aggressive form of cancer.

When I heard the diagnosis, all kinds of fears and thoughts raced through my mind. I asked about surgery and all of the alternatives. Considering my young age and the fact that the cancer appeared to be confined to the capsule of the prostate gland, my doctor recommended immediate surgery so the cancer wouldn't spread to the lymph nodes.

After talking it over with my wife and the owner of the team, I decided to go ahead and get it done. I had surgery on July 6, 1994, and the cancer was indeed confined to the gland; I didn't need any additional treatment. My last PSA test was 0.02, and today I am feeling great.

I think the real reason I was diagnosed is because as general manager of a professional baseball team, I can stand up on a soap box and help educate others about the importance of early detection and treatment. I can use my position to say that prostate cancer is a disease that will hit anyone from any walk of life. This is a disease that all men must acknowledge as a threat, and the best defense is education — through books such as these, through support groups, through talking to your doctor.

In my opinion, the most important message you'll find in this book is that if you're black and/or have a family history of prostate cancer, you need to start getting screened with BOTH the PSA blood test and the digital-rectal exam, or DRE, by age 40. My urologist told me that a digital exam alone would have probably missed my cancer for another couple of years, and with the kind of malignancy I had, a diagnosis by that time would have been too late.

If there's just one message I can leave with you, it is this: don't let a fear of the digital-rectal exam keep you from getting regular prostate checkups. The DRE and PSA tests are both quick and painless, and together they just may save your life.

After all, I'm living proof.

Bob Watson

General manager, New York Yankees

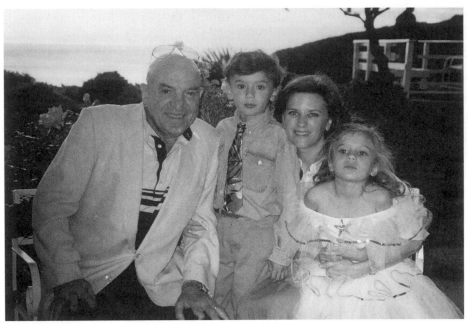

The late Telly Savalas with his wife, Julie, and their children.

To millions of people around the world, Telly Savalas was Kojak. To me, he was my charismatic husband. To his children, he was simply their dear, wonderful Papa.

When my husband passed away in January 1994, it was mistakenly reported that he had suffered from prostate cancer. The truth was that he had bladder cancer. As anyone who has witnessed the horror of cancer will tell you, it really doesn't matter what kind it is. It strikes terror in the hearts of us all. What a sad legacy this disease has wrought. It has united all of humanity with one frightening link. Very few of us have been spared the pain of knowing a loved one or friend afflicted with this disease and the hopeless despair that it invokes.

Yet for all the fear surrounding cancer, it is ignorance of the disease itself that we should be most afraid. That is why this book, as the title suggests, could indeed save your life or that of a loved one. Read it. Learn from it.

Because of fear, people tend to ignore the warning signs of cancer. Sadly, my husband was one of those people.

Telly was a man of great inner strength. He seemed invincible and was highly capable of dealing with whatever challenges life dealt him. Yet when he began having warning signs that something was amiss with his health, he chose to ignore them. He had witnessed his father die a horrible death from bladder cancer many, many years before when techniques and strategies for curing it were fairly archaic. Modern medicine had made huge strides in the treatment of bladder cancer, yet Telly was unable to let go of the memory of his father's suffering. It was because of this fear that he kept his symptoms to himself for more than three years. By the time he finally went to the doctor, he had lost so much blood while urinating that a blood transfusion was necessary. The doctors were angry and saddened by his inability to come to them sooner.

Bladder and prostate cancer are two of the most easily treatable of all cancers. Had my husband gone to the doctor when he first noticed the warning signs, he would still be here today. Fear and ignorance can be a fatal combination.

My children are 9 and 11 now. Their father passed away more than two years ago, and not a day goes by that they don't yearn for the sound of his voice or the reassuring warmth of his embrace. If only we could rewrite our story and create a happy ending. Unfortunately, that can only happen in the movies. In real life, we must write the script of our lives with great care. Our health decisions affect not only ourselves but all of those who love and need us.

Julie Savalas

Wife of late "Kojak" star Telly Savalas

1

Preparing for Your Prostate Checkup

A

Why should I know
about my prostate?

B

Can prostate cancer
be prevented?

C

When should I first have
my prostate examined?

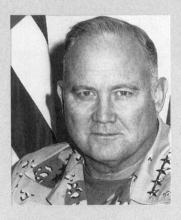

H. Norman Schwarzkopf
U.S. Army general, retired

The PSA test is important, but by itself it is not enough (my number was 1.2, which led me to believe I didn't have cancer). The digital-rectal examination is absolutely necessary and the patient should challenge the doctor to take as much time as is necessary for a thorough examination. Screening and early detection allowed me to undergo a complete cure, and today I am cancer-free.

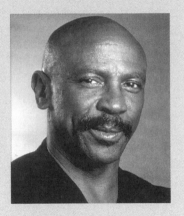

Lou Gossett Jr.
Actor

When an uncle died of prostate cancer, my family did not talk about the cause of his death; prostate cancer was a taboo topic back then. Fortunately today, with educational books like this, information about prostate cancer and prostate disease is easily available and easy to understand. Increased awareness and early detection is the key to winning the battle against prostate cancer. This disease can be beaten if caught early enough.

I do not have prostate cancer but I wanted to contribute to this book because this disease significantly affects the African-American community. African-American men are at least twice as likely to get prostate cancer than any other men. We need to get this message out there so increased awareness and early detection can become a priority.

A
Why should I know about my prostate?

First, you should know about your prostate gland because prostate cancer is common; it affects one in eight American men. Every three minutes a man is diagnosed with the disease, making it the most commonly detected malignancy in men today. In 1995, more than 244,000 new cases were diagnosed in the United States. In 1998, an estimated 400,000 Americans will get the news.

Second, you should know about your prostate because prostate cancer kills. It is the second most common cause of cancer death in men, next to lung cancer (see Table 1A). In 1990, nearly 32,500 Americans died of prostate cancer. In 1996, almost 41,000 will die of the disease — that's one man every 13 minutes.

Table 1A — The Top Three Types of Newly Diagnosed Cancer and the Top Three Causes of Cancer in 1996 for Men in the United States (by Body/Organ Site)

Most Common Cancer Cases In Men: 1996

Rank	Cancer Types	Percentage of All Cancer Cases
1	Prostate	41%
2	Lung	13%
3	Colon & rectal	9%

Most Common Cancer Deaths In Men: 1996

Rank	Cancer Types	Percentage of All Cancer Deaths
1	Lung	32%
2	Prostate	14%
3	Colon & rectal	9%

Source: *CA – Cancer Journal for Clinicians,* Volume 46(1), Pages 5-27, January-February 1996.

If current trends continue, there will be a 90-percent increase in the number of prostate cancers diagnosed and a 37-percent increase in prostate-cancer deaths by the year 2000 as compared with the 1980s.

So now you know that prostate cancer is a big public health problem. But what should you know about the prostate itself, apart from the fact that everyone agrees it is shaped like a walnut? Here are the basics:

Only men have a prostate. Being a gland, its purpose is to secrete about one-third of the fluid that carries sperm during ejaculation, or orgasm. (The rest of the fluid is secreted by the two seminal vesicles, which lie on opposite sides of the prostate. The sperm itself is produced by the testicles, which also make the male hormone testosterone.)

The prostate sits deep within the body, just below the bladder and above the rectum (see Fig. 1A). The gland has four major areas, or zones:

- **the peripheral zone** — the gland's largest zone, this is the part the doctor feels during a rectal exam and is the place where most prostate cancers begin to grow;
- **the transition zone** — where a noncancerous condition called benign prostatic hyperplasia, or BPH, occurs and where a small number of prostate cancers grow;
- **the central zone** — where an even smaller number of prostate cancers begin; and
- **the periurethral zone** — a tiny area where virtually no malignancies originate.

The prostate is surrounded by delicate structures such as blood vessels; a group of nerves responsible for erection; and the external sphincter, the primary muscle needed for urinary control. This muscle, which can be tightened voluntarily, is what allows a man to prevent his bladder from leaking even when it is uncomfortably full. The external sphincter should not be confused with another nearby muscle called the internal sphincter, which cannot be controlled at will. It tightens automatically, a function that allows the bladder to hold urine.

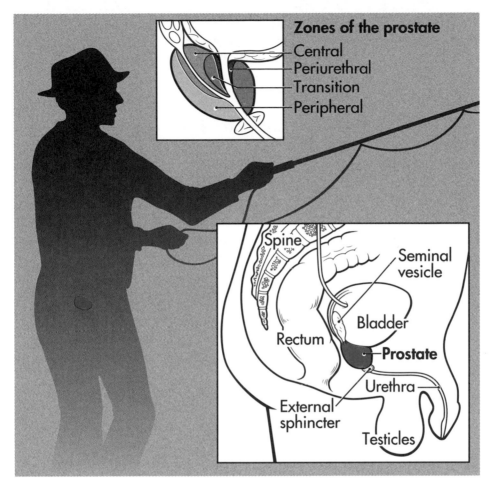

Zones of the prostate
- Central
- Periurethral
- Transition
- Peripheral

Spine

Seminal vesicle

Rectum

Bladder

Prostate

Urethra

External sphincter

Testicles

Fig. 1A — Anatomy of the Prostate Gland

- *The fisherman shows that the prostate is located deep within the pelvic area.*

- *The big box shows that the prostate is located below the bladder and next to the rectum.*

- *The small box shows that the prostate is divided into four areas (listed from largest to smallest): the peripheral zone, the transition zone, the central zone and the periurethral zone.*

Tunneling through the prostate is the urethra, the channel that carries urine and semen from the body. About 8 inches long, the urethra begins at the bottom of the bladder and ends at the tip of the penis; the prostate surrounds only about the first inch of the urethra.

The activity of the prostate is controlled by male hormones, called androgens, which provide the fuel that keeps the prostate running. One form of androgen is the male hormone testosterone. Cut off the supply of testosterone to the prostate and the gland can no longer function. Another, stronger, type of testosterone is called DHT (dihydrotestosterone), which the prostate also needs to function properly.

The prostate gets larger with age. This may be strange to imagine because most of the body stops growing soon after puberty. However, the prostate continues to grow throughout a man's life. When the prostate enlarges, it not only expands outward but also can grow inward, squeezing the urethra and causing urinary problems. Imagine that the prostate is an orange and the urethra is a straw running through it. Squeeze the orange, and the straw can no longer stay open and transfer fluid.

FAST FACT

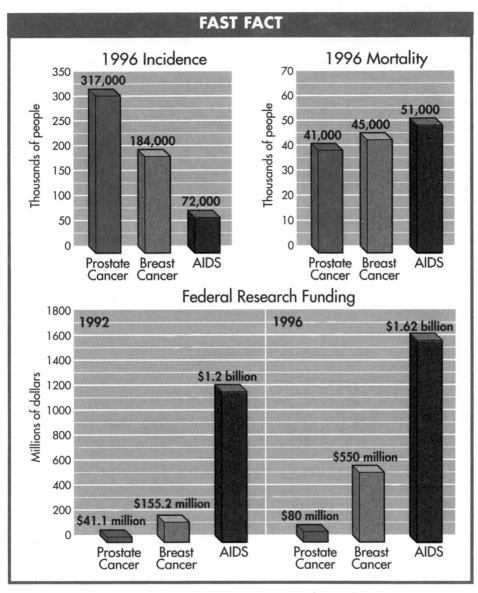

Source: American Foundation for Urologic Disease (AFUD).

B

Can prostate cancer be prevented?

Unfortunately, the major risk factors for prostate cancer cannot be prevented, such as age, race and family medical history. Fortunately, other factors that may increase one's chances of getting the disease can be controlled, from sun exposure to diet to occupation (see Table 1B-1).

Nonpreventable risk factors

Age — As a man gets older, his risk of developing prostate cancer increases significantly. Few men in their 20s or 30s are diagnosed with prostate cancer, but by age 50, almost 33 percent of men have small prostate tumors. By age 80 about 75 percent of men are believed to have prostate cancer, and by age 90, about 90 percent have the disease.

Race — Ethnic background plays a definite role in prostate-cancer risk. Blacks are about twice as likely to develop prostate cancer than members of any other race. Asians, on the other hand, have the lowest incidence of prostate cancer, while whites fall in between (see Table 1B-2).

Hormone levels — High levels of testosterone are associated with an increased risk of prostate cancer. For example, men who've had their testicles removed before puberty rarely develop prostate cancer. Research indicates that Asian men may have the lowest testosterone levels of any race, which may account for their lower prostate-cancer risk, while black men have the highest, which may account for their doubled risk. Men with lower levels of sex-hormone-binding globulin (SHBG) also seem to be at an increased risk. On the other hand, men with higher levels of estradiol (female hormone) seem to be at a decreased risk for developing prostate cancer. Finally, the hormone DHT (dihydrotestosterone), which was thought to increase prostate-cancer risk, is now believed to play an undefined role, according to a recent study from the Harvard School of Public Health.

Table 1B-1 — Nonpreventable and Preventable Factors that May Increase, Decrease or Have No Bearing on Prostate-cancer Risk

May Increase Your Risk	May Decrease Your Risk	Likely Has No Impact On Your Risk
Alcohol	Diet low in saturated fat, high in fiber	Bacterial or viral infection
Arsenic levels in well water	Exercise	Benign enlargement of the prostate (BPH)
Decreased levels of sex-hormone-binding globulin (SHBG)	Increased levels of estradiol (female hormone)	Beta carotene (a type of vitamin A)
Decreased ultraviolet light exposure or decreased amounts of vitamin D	Increased ultraviolet light exposure or increased amounts of vitamin D	Family history of other cancers
Diet high in saturated fat and low in fiber	Selenium	Frequency of sexual intercourse
Family history of prostate cancer	Soy products	Income level
Increasing age	Tomatoes (lycopene)	Most occupations
Increased levels of testosterone	Tea	Number of sexual partners
Race (black)		Prostatitis (prostate infection)
Some occupations (water treatment; aircraft manufacturing; railway transport; power, gas and water utilities; farming; fishing; and forestry)		Religion
Some occupational exposures (metallic dust, liquid fuel combustion products, lubricating oils and greases, poly-aromatic hydrocarbons from coal, rare elements such as tritium, 51Cr, 59Fe, 60Co or 65Zn, or large amounts of herbicides and pesticides)		Sexually transmitted diseases
		Smoking
		Vasectomy*

*The National Institutes of Health recently reviewed all of the data on vasectomy and concluded that this sterilization procedure does not increase one's risk of getting prostate cancer. The small risk that did surface in a few studies was explained by the fact that most vasectomies are done by urologists, whose patients are more likely to get their prostates checked regularly.

Table 1B-2 — The Percentage of Deaths Due to Prostate Cancer in the United States According to Race and Ethnicity

Race and Ethnicity	Percentage of Deaths Due to Prostate Cancer
Blacks	9.4%
Whites	6.3%
Native Americans	5.9%
Hispanics	5.7%
Asians and Pacific Islanders	3.9%

Source: *CA – Cancer Journal for Clinicians,* Volume 46(1), Pages 5-27, January-February 1996.

Family history — In the United States, the average man's risk of getting prostate cancer is between 10 percent and 15 percent. The greater number of family members who have had the disease, the higher the risk of not only getting prostate cancer but developing it earlier. If a single family member has had prostate cancer, the risk is double. If two family members have had prostate cancer, the risk becomes two to five times higher. It doesn't matter whether the prostate cancer comes from the mother's or father's side of the family; the risk is the same.

Other types of cancer within the family (such as breast, colon, endometrial or ovarian) have not been strongly linked to prostate-cancer risk, although the possible causes of many of these cancers are thought to be related.

Preventable risk factors

Environment — In China and Japan, only a small number of men die of prostate cancer each year. But once a Chinese or Japanese man moves to the United States, his risk of dying from prostate cancer increases to become nearly comparable to that of the average American male. This is just one example of the general rule that when men move to another country, as time goes by, they come close to achieving the prostate-cancer risk of that nation. The pos-

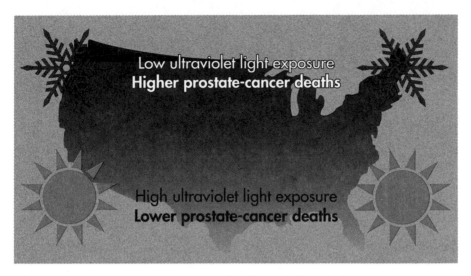

Fig. 1B — Prostate Cancer and Ultraviolet Light

The risk of death from prostate cancer is influenced by sun exposure. In the North, men are exposed to less sun and have a greater risk of dying from prostate cancer. In the South, men are exposed to more sun and thus have a lesser risk of dying from the disease. This implies that ultraviolet light exposure may help prevent prostate cancer.

sible environmental or genetic factors that contribute to this phenomenon are not fully understood, but a variety of possible clues are emerging.

Sun exposure is one such clue. In the United States, for example, men living in the South have a smaller chance of dying from prostate cancer than men living in the North (see Fig. 1B). The theory is that exposure to ultraviolet radiation from the sun has a protective effect against prostate cancer. This may be true, because ultraviolet radiation activates production of vitamin D in the body, which has been known to have some anti-cancer effects. In fact, the largest source of vitamin D comes from exposure to ultraviolet light. This may help explain why prostate-cancer death rates are highest in areas with less exposure to the sun's ultraviolet rays, such as Scandinavia and North America or especially polluted Northern cities.

This sun-exposure theory also may explain why black men — even those who live in Southern climates — are about twice as likely to develop prostate cancer as anyone else, for their highly pigmented skin absorbs less ultraviolet radiation and thus their bodies produce less vitamin D. In addition, for reasons not fully understood, black men have a greater chance of not only developing prostate cancer but developing it at an earlier age than other men in general.

While the body's largest source of vitamin D comes from ultraviolet light, you do not want to drastically increase your sun exposure because of the risk of skin cancer. But it would not hurt to get more vitamin D in your diet (but please stay within the recommended daily allowance; too much vitamin D in the diet can also lead to side effects) or to spend a little more time outdoors. As the old saying goes, "everything in moderation."

Diet — A diet high in saturated fat (especially animal fat) and low in fiber strongly increases the risk of prostate cancer. Animal studies have shown that prostate tumors grow faster in animals fed a high-fat diet. People who live in Asia eat less fat than Americans and they consume larger quantities of fish (a good source of vitamin D), which may be a partial explanation for the lower incidence of death from prostate cancer in China and Japan. While beta carotene (a cancer-preventive nutrient found in orange-colored foods) has not been shown to decrease prostate-cancer risk, lycopene (a pigment found in fresh tomatoes and tomato sauce) has been shown to lower such risk.

Occupation — Industries such as water treatment; aircraft manufacturing; railway transport; power, gas and water utilities; farming; fishing and forestry have been associated with prostate-cancer risk, but the evidence so far leans only toward a slight or possible association. The slight increase for farmers may be due to an increased exposure to pesticides. Other occupational exposures, such as Agent Orange, have not been studied.

FAST FACT

The risk of getting prostate cancer rises with the amount of alcohol consumed. According to a recent study, men who have 22 or more alcoholic drinks per week increase their risk of getting prostate cancer.

c

When should I first have
my prostate examined?

When you should begin getting annual prostate exams depends upon your risk of getting prostate cancer. We have provided examples of two prostate-cancer risk trees: one with a strong family history of prostate cancer that calls for starting prostate checkups at age 40, and one without a family background of prostate cancer that calls for beginning annual exams at age 50 (see Fig. 1C-1). To help determine your risk, the first thing you should do is find out if anyone in your family has had prostate cancer and then fill out the family prostate-cancer risk tree provided in this book (see Fig. 1C-2).

If possible, trace all of the men in your family back to your grandfathers on each side. List their respective ages, if they are alive, and whether they were diagnosed with and/or died of prostate cancer. If you are not absolutely certain of the information, put down your best guess with a question mark next to it. It is important to list not only what your male family members died of, but what other health problems they may have had. For example, it would be important to know that a family member who'd been diagnosed with prostate cancer actually died some years later of heart problems. This would indicate an increased risk of prostate cancer and a possible risk of heart disease. Finally, it would not hurt to list, at the bottom of the page or on another sheet of paper, your male and female family members who have had cancer. Although there is not a strong risk of getting prostate cancer if your family has a history of other cancers, this additional information could assist your doctor in giving you the best possible medical care in the future.

After you have some knowledge of your family's prostate-cancer history, you and your health care provider can determine whether you should begin having annual prostate exams at age 40 or 50, depending on your risk of getting the disease.

Those who should start yearly prostate exams by AGE 40:

- black men with a life expectancy of at least 10 years
- men with a family history of prostate cancer on either side of their family who are expected to live at least 10 more years

Those who should start annual prostate exams by AGE 50:

- men with no family history of prostate cancer who have a life expectancy of at least 10 years

If you are extremely concerned about prostate cancer or if you believe there's a history of the disease in your family but are not certain how some of your male relatives have died, then you should begin getting yearly prostate exams at age 40 just to be safe.

Men who are expected to live at least 10 more years will benefit the most from early detection of prostate cancer. Because prostate cancer is usually a slow-growing malignancy, older men or younger individuals with a life expectancy of less than 10 years will probably die of something else, so early detection may not be of benefit to them.

Your chances of getting prostate cancer can be even more accurately determined if any of your family members were diagnosed with the disease (see Table 1C).

When should you discontinue your annual prostate exams? This depends on your current health status and family health history. For example, the average male life expectancy in the United States is 83 years. So if you are 68 years old, in good health and have a number of relatives who have lived beyond age 80, there is no reason why you shouldn't continue to get checked annually, at least until your early 70s. Ultimately, the decision of when to cease such exams is made together by you and your doctor.

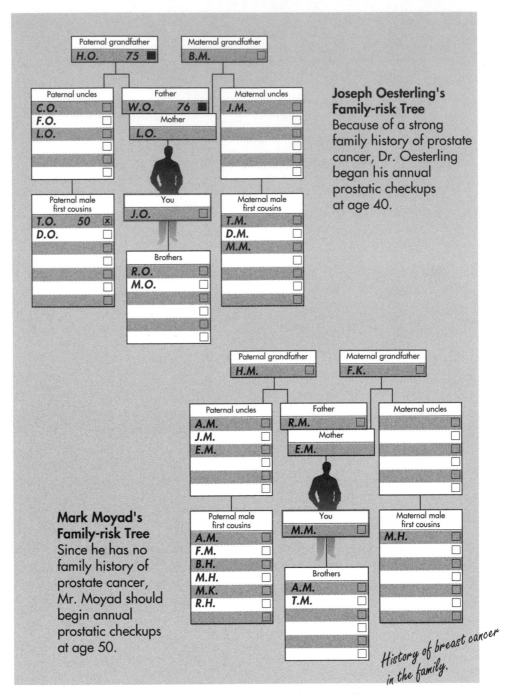

Joseph Oesterling's Family-risk Tree
Because of a strong family history of prostate cancer, Dr. Oesterling began his annual prostatic checkups at age 40.

Mark Moyad's Family-risk Tree
Since he has no family history of prostate cancer, Mr. Moyad should begin annual prostatic checkups at age 50.

History of breast cancer in the family.

Fig. 1C-1 — Two Samples of Family-risk Trees for Prostate Cancer: High Risk (Top) and Low Risk (Bottom)

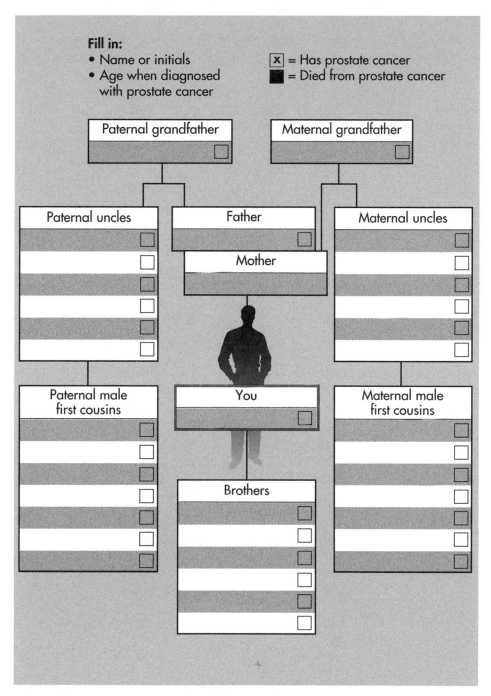

Fig. 1C-2 — Your Family-risk Tree for Prostate Cancer

For you to copy, fill out and share with your doctor.

Table 1C — Every man in the United States has a 13-percent risk of getting prostate cancer and a 3-percent chance of dying from it. However, one's risk increases with the number of family members who've had the disease.

Relatives Diagnosed with Prostate Cancer	Percentage of Men in This Situation Who Get Prostate Cancer
No (zero) relatives diagnosed with prostate cancer	13%
A grandfather	20%
Your father	26%
An uncle	20%
A cousin	16%
A brother	26%
Two brothers	65%
Your grandfather & father	about 100%
Your grandfather, father & a brother	about 100%

Source: *Journal of Urology*, Volume 150, Pages 797-802, September 1993.

FAST FACT

Between 5 percent and 10 percent of all prostate cancers are due to genetics (family history), while an equal number are due to environmental factors (alcohol, diet, sunlight exposure). The other 80 percent to 90 percent of cases are due to a combination of genetics and environment.

The ABCs of CHAPTER 1
A Quick Review

A
Why should I know about my prostate?

- Prostate cancer is common; it affects one man in eight.
- Prostate cancer kills; it is the second most common cause of cancer deaths in men, claiming 40,000 lives each year.
- As the prostate gets larger with age, it may squeeze the urethra and cause urinary problems.

B
Can prostate cancer be prevented?

- Factors that decrease prostate-cancer risk include a low-fat, high-fiber diet.
- Black men and those with a family history of prostate cancer (on either side) have a greater chance of getting the disease.

- Factors that have no known significant influence on prostate-cancer risk include benign prostatic hyperplasia (BPH), smoking and vasectomy.

C
When should I first have my prostate examined?

- Investigate your family's disease history and discuss it with your doctor to help determine when you should begin getting your prostate examined.
- Your yearly prostate exams should begin at age 40 if you are black or if you have a history of prostate cancer in your family (presuming you have a life expectancy of at least 10 years).
- Your yearly prostate exams should begin at age 50 if you have no known family history of prostate cancer and are expected to live at least 10 more years.

Medical References

Title: **"Cancer Statistics, 1996"**
Authors: Parker, S.L.; Tong, T.; Bolden, S.; et al
Journal: *CA — Cancer Journal for Clinicians*
Volume: 46 (1)
Pages: 5-27
Date: January-February 1996

Title: **"A prospective study of dietary fat and risk of prostate cancer"**
Authors: Giovannucci, E.; Rimm, E.B.; Colditz, G.A.; et al
Journal: *Journal of the National Cancer Institute*
Volume: 85 (19)
Pages: 1571-1579
Date: Oct. 6, 1993

Title: **"Hereditary prostate cancer: epidemiologic and clinical features"**
Authors: Carter, B.S.; Bova, G.S.; Beaty, T.H.; et al
Journal: *Journal of Urology*
Volume: 150 (3)
Pages: 797-802
Date: September 1993

Title: **"Geographic patterns of prostate cancer mortality"**
Authors: Hanchette, C.L.; and Schwartz, G.G.
Journal: *Cancer*
Volume: 70 (12)
Pages: 2861-2869
Date: Dec. 15, 1992

Title: **"Occupational risk factors for prostate cancer: Results from a case-control study in Montreal, Quebec, Canada"**
Authors: Aronson, K.J.; Siemiatycki, J.; Dewar, R.; and Gerin, M.
Journal: *American Journal of Epidemiology*
Volume: 143(4)
Pages: 363-373
Date: Feb. 15, 1996

2

What to Expect During a Prostate Exam

A

What kind of doctor performs
this type of exam?

B

Is a digital-rectal exam really necessary?
What about the PSA blood test?

C

My test results are abnormal.
What do I do next?

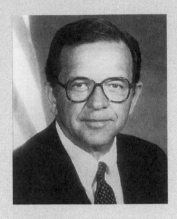

**Ted Stevens
U.S. senator**

An annual prostate checkup meant much for me. My physician found signs of change in my prostate during my yearly visit in 1990. After follow-up tests, the diagnosis was cancer — before it had spread. Surgery took care of my problem; annual exams continue to confirm complete recovery.

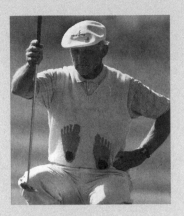

**Jim Ferree
Senior professional golfer**

Thanks to the PSA test in 1991 that led to the early detection of my prostate cancer, I am still playing competitive golf on the Senior PGA Tour. Without the early detection, I might now be looking up at the grass instead of playing on it.

A

What kind of doctor performs this type of exam?

So you are ready to have your prostate examined. However, you may not have a regular physician or if you do, you are not certain whether she/he is qualified to perform a prostate checkup. Who should you ask for?

The prostate exam (see Table 2A) is performed by three types of physicians: the oncologist, the primary care doctor and the urologist (see Fig. 2A).

Table 2A — The Tests Used for a Prostate Exam and the Meaning of Their Results

The Test	What is Normal?	What is Abnormal?*
Digital-rectal exam (also called a DRE)	Prostate size is small	Prostate size is large
	Prostate feels smooth, symmetrical and elastic	Prostate consistency is rough, asymmetric and hard
	Prostate anatomical borders can be felt, without feeling non-prostate structures	Prostate anatomical borders are hard, and the seminal vesicles can be felt
Prostate-specific antigen (also called PSA)	0-4 ng/ml	Greater than 4 ng/ml
Ultrasound (also called a transrectal ultrasound, or TRUS)	No darker-than-normal (hypoechoic) areas; prostate appears uniform (homogenous) throughout, with distinct borders; neighboring structures observable (bladder, rectum, seminal vesicles)	Hypoechoic (darker than normal) area within the prostate gland

*not necessarily cancerous

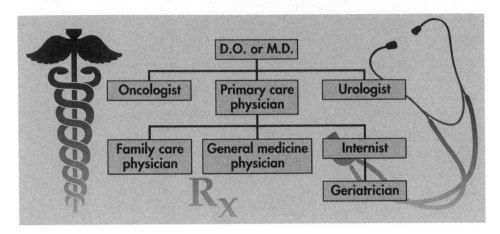

Fig. 2A — Doctors Who Perform a Prostate Checkup

There are two types of doctors: the doctor of osteopathic medicine (D.O.) and the doctor of medicine (M.D.), both of whom can perform the prostate exam. There are three types of D.O.s and M.D.s who are qualified to do this exam: the oncologist (cancer doctor), the primary care physician (a specialist in family medicine, general medicine, internal medicine or geriatrics) and the urologist (a specialist in disorders of the urinary tract).

The oncologist — This type of doctor specializes in cancer treatment, but she/he is also qualified to perform a prostate checkup.

The primary care doctor — There are four types of primary care doctors who perform prostate exams: the family doctor, who may also be called a family care doctor or family practice doctor; the internist (not to be confused with an intern, who is a doctor in training), who may also be called an internal medicine doctor; a general medicine doctor, who can be qualified as a family practice and/or internal medicine doctor; and a geriatrician, who treats older individuals and who may also be found in the internal medicine category of the Yellow Pages or hospital directory.

The urologist — This type of doctor specializes in disorders of the urinary tract, such as problems with the kidneys, bladder, prostate and testicles.

There also may be some confusion as to what type of degree the doctor should have. There are osteopathic doctors, or D.O.s, and medical doctors, or M.D.s, in the above three specialties. Doctors of osteopathic medicine and medical doctors go through a similar educational process, so both are equally qualified to perform a prostate checkup, regardless of whether they specialize in oncology, primary care or urology.

Regardless of which type of physician performs your annual prostate checkup, it should always be the same doctor or a doctor from the same group, if possible. Staying within the same practice is important because doctors who work together have better access to each other's patient records.

If you move or travel frequently, it is important to remember that when you get a prostate checkup, you should have your regular doctor provide a written report about your current and previous checkups (some individuals keep a copy of their own medical records) so that it can be shared with your new or temporary doctor. This way, your new physician will have this valuable information and you will continue to get the most out of your office visits.

What if you don't have any medical insurance but need a prostate checkup? You should feel free to call various doctors offices and walk-in clinics and ask what they charge for such an exam, and you should pick the physician who charges the least. You also could call your local public health unit, which may charge little or nothing for the exam. In addition, some hospitals or medical centers periodically provide free prostate exams throughout the year, as during national Prostate Cancer Awareness Week, which is usually the third week of September.

FAST FACT

More than four out of every 10 men (40 percent) diagnosed with prostate cancer will have metastatic disease (cancer that has spread beyond the prostate). Symptoms of localized prostate cancer are rare; warning signs don't usually appear until the cancer has escaped the prostate.

B

Is a digital-rectal exam really necessary? What about the PSA blood test?

The rectal exam is worthwhile and necessary because it could save your life!

The rectal exam is also known as the digital-rectal examination, or DRE. During this procedure, the doctor's index finger (digit) is inserted into the rectum to feel for any suspicious changes on the surface of the prostate. The index finger is used because it is the most sensitive finger on the hand. The rectum is thin and flexible enough so that the prostate can be easily felt, much like a golf ball through a piece of wax paper. Usually only half of the doctor's index finger is needed to feel the gland, but this depends on the patient's weight. The heavier the man, the more of the index finger is inserted during the exam.

The rectal exam is simple to perform. The doctor will first ask you to put on a hospital robe/gown or you may just be asked to drop your pants and then position yourself in one of several ways, depending on which position your doctor thinks is most effective. The doctor may ask you to stand next to the examining table and bend forward a little, you may be asked to kneel on the examining table, or you may be asked to lie on your side (in a fetal position). All of these positions make it easier for the doctor's gloved and lubricated index finger to go past your anus and into your rectum so the prostate can be felt (see Fig. 2B).

The rectal exam itself is very quick, about five seconds. It may feel strange, but it should not be painful. If it is painful, tell your doctor, because it could be a sign of a prostate disorder such as prostatitis, or inflammation of the prostate.

The exam is also safe; if performed correctly, there is little to no chance of rectal injury. It also costs very little — just the price of a latex glove, some lubricant and a few seconds of the doctor's time.

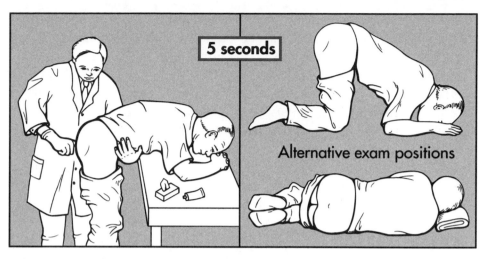

5 seconds

Alternative exam positions

Fig. 2B — The Digital-rectal Prostate Examination

The rectal exam itself takes about five seconds and can be performed at least three different ways: by having the patient stand and lean over the examining table (left); by having the patient kneel face-down on top of the examining table (top right); or by having the patient lie on his side, curled into a fetal position on top of the table (bottom right).

The reason the rectal exam is so necessary and can save your life is because most prostate cancers begin in an area of the prostate called the "peripheral zone," which can only be felt through this type of exam. Therefore the rectal exam can detect localized cancer — cancer that has not spread beyond the prostate — and current treatments can potentially cure this type of cancer.

If you are scared or embarrassed to have a rectal exam, please remember that your doctor has probably performed hundreds or even thousands of these tests. This is a routine exam for your doctor and there is no reason to feel embarrassed. Also, try and remember that you are doing something that could easily prevent an early death. Isn't this some of the same thinking you use to motivate yourself to eat right, exercise, decrease your amount of stress or maybe stop smoking?

Another test used with the rectal exam is the prostate-specific anti-gen, or PSA, blood test. PSA is secreted by the prostate whether the gland is normal or cancerous, but high levels of PSA in the blood-stream can mean that you have prostate cancer. The PSA test is simple; about a tablespoon of blood is taken from your arm with a needle, and the sample is sent to a laboratory where the PSA level is measured. The result is usually back within 24 hours. A normal PSA range is usually from 0 to 4 ng/ml (nanograms per milliliter). There are exceptions to this range, depending on your age and race (see Chapter 3). For example, because the prostate enlarges with age, it is normal for the gland to secrete more PSA as you get older. If your PSA level goes beyond 4 ng/ml, however, this means that you could have prostate cancer, even though the doctor may not feel anything suspicious during the rectal exam. This is why a prostate checkup should always include a rectal exam and a PSA blood test, because when used together, the chance of finding cancer is much better (see Table 2B). In addition, some doctors also use the ultra-sound test to detect prostate cancer, but it is not as reliable and accurate as the DRE or the PSA blood test together.

Table 2B — The Chances of Having Prostate Cancer Based On the Results of the Digital-rectal Exam (DRE) and the Prostate-specific Antigen (PSA) Blood Test

	PSA < 4 ng/ml	PSA 4-10 ng/ml	PSA > 10 ng/ml
Negative DRE	4-9 %	20-25 %	31-42 %
Positive DRE	10-17 %	41-62 %	67-77 %

There is controversy about the accuracy of the PSA test when doing annual checkups (see Chapter 3); therefore, some oncologists, pri-mary care doctors, or urologists may only perform the rectal exam. However, based on all the data available today, the PSA test should be a part of the checkup because it detects twice as many cancers as the rectal exam. Many of these are curable cancers that are still confined to the prostate. You have a right to request the PSA test or find another doctor who will provide one. The American Cancer Society, the American Urological Association and the American College of Radiology recommend the PSA test as part of the annual checkup for prostate cancer.

If your PSA and rectal exam are normal, then you are finished with this checkup and should come back for another in a year. If your PSA and/or rectal exam are abnormal, you will need additional testing.

FAST FACT

Zone of the Prostate	Percentage of Prostate Cancers That Begin There
Peripheral Zone	70%
(Part or most of this zone can be felt during the rectal exam and most of the biopsy is taken from here)	
Transitional Zone	20-25%
(This is the only zone where BPH occurs and some doctors take a biopsy from here)	
Central Zone	5-10%
Periuretheal Zone	0%

The four zones of the prostate and the percentage of prostate cancers that occur in each. Most cancers occur in the peripheral zone, which is the area of the prostate that can be felt during a digital-rectal exam. However, two-thirds of peripheral-zone cancers are too small to be detected during a DRE.

C

My test results are abnormal. What do I do next?

If either your PSA test or rectal exam are abnormal, your doctor will order several more tests (see Table 2C).

One such test is the transrectal ultrasound, or TRUS. This procedure involves a machine that uses sound waves to detect the difference between cancerous and noncancerous prostate tissue. You may know about ultrasound through its widespread use in pregnancy. It is used to see if the fetus is normal, and it can be used to determine the sex of an unborn baby. For a pregnant woman, the ultrasound transducer is placed on the belly. For a man having a prostate checkup, an ultrasound probe is placed inside the rectum, hence the name "transrectal" ultrasound. TRUS feels strange but it is painless, just like the rectal exam.

Table 2C — The Next Step After the Prostate Checkup

The Digital-rectal Exam (DRE) Result	The PSA Test Result	What the Doctor Should Say After Seeing the Results
Normal	Normal	"Come back in one year for another DRE and PSA."
Abnormal Normal Abnormal	Normal Abnormal Abnormal	"You need a transrectal ultrasound (TRUS)-guided biopsy with a total of at least six biopsy specimens (called a sextant biopsy)."

The doctor also will order a prostate biopsy. A biopsy is the removal and examination of a small piece of tissue from an area of the body that the doctor is concerned about, such as the prostate.

A prostate biopsy is performed under the guidance of TRUS, in which the sound waves from the rectal ultrasound probe act as a navigator to let the doctor accurately locate the prostate for tissue sampling. A tiny needle is then inserted alongside the probe to remove a small sample of prostate tissue, about 1/25th of an inch thick (see Fig. 2C-1). Usually a minimum of six individual pieces of tissue (called a sextant biopsy) are taken from different areas around the peripheral zone of the prostate (the area where three of every four cancers begin to grow). Some doctors also take two additional tissue samples from the transition zone of the prostate, because one in four prostate cancers begin there. The biopsies are then sent to a pathologist, which is a doctor who specializes in diagnosing cancer or other abnormalities from tissue samples. After a few days, you will hear one of the following results (see Fig. 2C-2):

The biopsy is negative — This means there is no cancer and you should come back in a year for another checkup.

The biopsy is in the "gray zone" — This indicates a condition called prostatic intraepithelial neoplasia, or PIN. If you are found to have PIN, it means your prostate cells look neither normal nor cancerous; their appearance falls somewhere in between — in the "gray zone." PIN is classified by grade: low (PIN I), or high (PIN II or III). The higher the grade of anything in medicine, the more aggressive something usually is. When low-grade PIN is diagnosed, there is no need for additional testing, and you are asked to come back in a year for your regular prostate exam. If you are found to have high-grade PIN (PIN II or III), you must return in four to six weeks for a repeat biopsy. Studies show that half of the men who have high-grade PIN upon the first biopsy will have cancer upon the repeat biopsy. Remember, this only applies to high-grade PIN, not the low-grade variety.

The biopsy is positive — This means there is cancer, and you need to talk to your doctor about treatment options (see Chapter 5).

After a biopsy, in a small number of cases you may have some blood in your urine, in your semen or you may bleed a little from the rectum. To prevent such bleeding, you will be told to stop using any products that may thin your blood, such as aspirin or the anticoagulant drug warfarin (brand name Coumadin) from three to 10 days beforehand, depending on the drug. These medications can be resumed the day after the biopsy.

There is very little pain involved with prostate biopsy because the needle is so tiny. Usually you do not need anesthesia or sedation during the procedure or any type of pain medication afterward. Also, the risk of infection is very low. This is because you are usually given an enema (a fluid solution used to flush out the lower intestine) the night before the biopsy, which cleans out the rectum and reduces the chance of infection. You are also given antibiotics before and after the biopsy to help prevent infection. You may also be asked to urinate before and after the biopsy so your doctor knows for sure that you did not experience any urinary complications from the procedure.

FAST FACT

Adenosis is a noncancerous condition of the prostate that can look like a low-grade cancer upon biopsy. The condition is found in about 1 percent of prostate biopsies. It usually occurs in the transition zone of the prostate, where benign prostatic hyperplasia, or BPH, occurs. Up to 20 percent of men surgically treated for BPH are found to have adenosis. If you have adenosis, do not worry. It is not cancer, and it is not an indication that you may get prostate cancer.

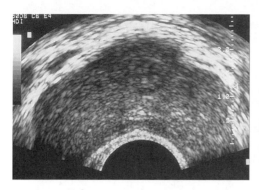

Normal (negative) ultrasound

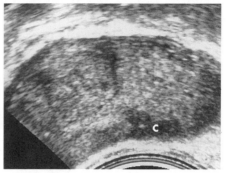

Abnormal (positive) ultrasound
(The "C" represents cancer)

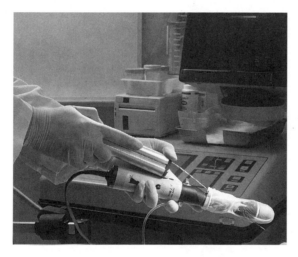

Fig. 2C-1 — Transrectal Ultrasound of the Prostate

The transrectal ultrasound (TRUS)-guided biopsy device (bottom), and examples of a normal and abnormal prostate ultrasound (top left and right).

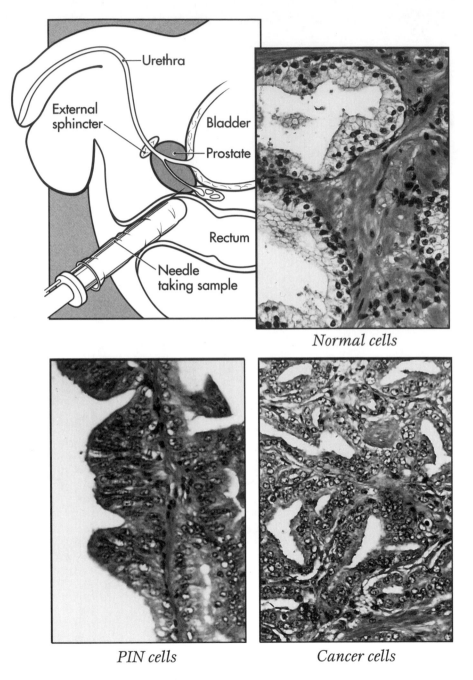

Normal cells

PIN cells

Cancer cells

Fig. 2C-2 — Prostate Biopsy

The biopsy procedure itself (top left) and the three types of prostate cells that can be found: normal, "gray zone" (PIN) or cancerous.

The ABCs of CHAPTER 2

A Quick Review

A

What kind of doctor performs this type of exam?

- A doctor of osteopathy (D.O.) or a medical doctor (M.D.) can perform a prostate exam. The doctor practices in one of the following specialties: oncology, primary care (family medicine, internal medicine, general medicine or geriatrics) or urology.

- Try to have the same doctor perform your exam every year, and if you move, have your doctor's office send all of your previous prostate exam information to your new doctor's office.

- If you do not have medical insurance or cannot afford the cost of a prostate exam, check with local hospitals, clinics, and public health units to see whether they may offer the checkup for free or for a reduced price at certain times of the year.

B

Is a digital-rectal exam really necessary? What about the PSA blood test?

- A prostate checkup consists of a rectal exam and a PSA test.

- If your rectal exam and PSA are normal, then you are finished with your checkup and should return in a year.

- If your rectal exam and/or PSA are abnormal, then you need a transrectal ultrasound (TRUS)-guided biopsy.

C

My test results are abnormal. What do I do next?

- If the biopsy is negative or indicates a low-grade form of prostatic intraepithelial neoplasia (also called PIN I), this means there is no cancer and you should come back in a year for your annual checkup.

- If the biopsy indicates high-grade PIN (also called PIN II or PIN III), this means that you are in the "gray area" of prostate-cancer detection and will have to return for a repeat biopsy in four to six weeks. Studies show that half of the men who have high-grade PIN are found to have cancer upon repeat biopsy.

- If the biopsy is positive and there is cancer, you and your doctor will need to discuss your treatment options (see Chapter 5).

Medical References

Title: **"Prostatic intraepithelial neoplasia is a risk factor for adenocarcinoma: predictive accuracy in needle biopsies"**
Authors: Davidson, D.; Bostwick, D.G.; Oesterling, J.E.; et al
Journal: *Journal of Urology*
Volume: 154 (4)
Pages: 1295-1299
Date: October 1995

Title: **"Prostate-specific antigen, digital-rectal examination, and transrectal ultrasonography: their roles in diagnosing prostate cancer"**
Authors: Cupp, M.R.; and Oesterling, J.E.
Journal: *Mayo Clinic Proceedings*
Volume: 68
Pages: 297-306
Date: March 1993

Title: **"Prostate-specific antigen: improving its ability to diagnose early prostate cancer"**
Author: Oesterling, J.E.
Journal: *Journal of the American Medical Association (JAMA)*
Volume: 267

Pages: 2236-2238
Date: April 22-29, 1992

Title: **"Ultrasound guided transrectal core biopsies of the palpably abnormal prostate"**
Authors: Hodge, K.K.; McNeal, J.E.; and Stamey, T.A.
Journal: *Journal of Urology*
Volume: 142 (1)
Pages: 66-70
Date: July 1989

Title: **"Clinical application of transrectal ultrasonography and prostate-specific antigen in the search for prostate cancer"**
Authors: Cooner, W.H.; Mosley B.R.; Rutherford, C.L. Jr.; et al
Journal: *Journal of Urology*
Volume: 139 (4)
Pages: 758-761
Date: April 1988

3

The PSA Blood Test for Prostate Cancer:

What You Need to Know

A

What is PSA? How do I understand my PSA test result?
Why is there controversy about this test?

B

What factors could affect my PSA level?

C

Are all PSA tests created equal?

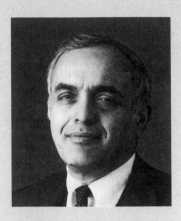

Robert D. Novak
Broadcast journalist

It astonishes me that there are so many complaints about the use of PSA testing and radical surgery, or prostatectomy. To wit:

• PSA can produce false negatives. *So what? Isn't it better to have some false alarms (that are disproved by subsequent tests) than die of cancer? In my case and in thousands of others, it was surely no false positive.*

• Prostate operations on elderly gentlemen, even when successful, often do not prolong their lives much longer. *This is a numbers game. Of course, many men die soon after a prostatectomy — but not from prostate cancer.*

• The ill effects of prostate surgery can be worse than the disease. *Not when a skilled surgeon is wielding the scalpel. My life has not been changed by surgery, but it has been prolonged.*

More medical research is needed to improve cure, detection and — ultimately — prevention. But for now the answer is to stop the petty grousing and work toward the universal administration of PSA tests.

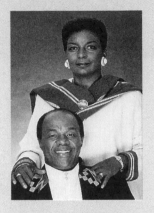

Marion Barry
Mayor, Washington, D.C.

I was diagnosed with prostate cancer on Oct. 13, 1995 — the weekend of the Million Man March. I didn't want to tell my wife, because she was very involved with the march and I didn't want to upset her. So I waited until the following week to tell her.

My wife was devastated and my friends were sympathetic. But I found that a lot of the people I talked to didn't know much about prostate cancer, just like I didn't know much about it. I was ignorant about this subject, I really was. For example, my first PSA test was in 1994, when I was 58. Quite frankly, I knew nothing about PSA; nobody had ever told me it was something you ought to look at.

The best advice I can give is to get a yearly prostate examination; African-American men should start when they're age 40. And if you do get the diagnosis, don't panic, because most men can be cured with the right treatment if their cancer is caught early enough. I chose surgery, and today my PSA is 0.

Marion Barry and his wife, Cora Masters-Barry, above.

A

What is PSA?
How do I understand my PSA test result?
Why is there controversy about this test?

Prostate-specific antigen, or PSA, is an enzyme produced by the prostate. Large quantities of PSA are found in the semen, which is released during ejaculation, or orgasm.

In younger men, PSA is not normally present in the bloodstream in large amounts. However, because the prostate gland enlarges with age, it is normal for older men to have slightly more PSA in their circulation because their prostates produce more of this product.

In addition to age-related prostate enlargement (a condition called benign prostatic hyperplasia, or BPH), another noncancerous condition that can cause PSA levels to rise is prostatitis, or infection and inflammation of the prostate. While BPH and prostatitis can cause PSA levels to inch upward, prostate cancer usually causes a more dramatic rise. However, about one in four prostate cancers do not cause an elevation in PSA. This is why the PSA blood test is not perfect and is part of the reason why its use has been controversial.

The standard normal range for PSA in the bloodstream is 0-4 ng/ml (nanograms per milliliter). When a reading falls between 4-10 ng/ml, interpretation can become difficult. A test result within this so-called "gray zone" could indeed be normal for that individual or could indicate a variety of conditions, including cancer.

The discovery that PSA tends to rise with age has led to the widespread use of "age-specific reference ranges" for determining normal PSA levels. While the first studies were based on white men, recent separate studies with Asian and black men have found that normal PSA values differ slightly between the races (see Table 3A).

Table 3A — Age-specific PSA Reference Ranges for Asians, Blacks and Whites

The greatest difference between the races occurs among men in their 50s and 70s. Age-specific reference ranges have not yet been determined for men age 80 and above.

Age Range	PSA Reference Ranges		
	Asians	Blacks	Whites
40-49	0-2.0	0-2.0	0-2.5
50-59	0-3.0	0-4.0	0-3.5
60-69	0-4.0	0-4.5	0-4.5
70-79	0-5.0	0-5.5	0-6.5

So although the traditional normal PSA range is between 0-4 ng/ml, the upper limit of normal can be as low as 2 ng/ml or as high as 6.5 ng/ml, depending on a man's age and race.

Age-specific references ranges have increased the detection of prostate cancers in younger men (those under 60) and eliminated prostate biopsies in older men (those over 60), making PSA a more accurate and clinically useful test for diagnosing prostate cancer.

Regardless of age and race, however, PSA levels greater than 10 ng/ml are a pretty accurate sign of prostate cancer; research shows that 70 percent to 80 percent of those who have a test result this high (also with a positive digital-rectal exam) are found to have the disease.

But even if the numbers are frightening, a PSA test, alone or in combination with a digital-rectal exam, only indicates there might be a problem; a prostate biopsy is always needed to confirm the presence of cancer.

The PSA assay by itself, just like any other blood test, is not perfect. As a result, researchers are looking into new methods of interpreting PSA values to improve the test's accuracy:

PSA density — Also called PSAD, this is a measurement technique in which the concentration of PSA in the blood is divided by the volume, or size, of the prostate gland, as measured by transrectal ultrasound. If this number, called PSA density, is greater than 0.15 and the PSA value is between 4-10 ng/ml, then a biopsy is recommended. However, the use of PSA density in prostate-cancer screening is questionable. Many doctors who use age-specific PSA reference ranges do not bother to calculate the PSA density because they feel it is of no extra benefit. In general, the age-specific ranges provide as much information as PSA density and eliminate the need for a transrectal ultrasound.

PSA velocity — Also called PSAV and PSA slope, this interpretation method takes into account the change in PSA level over time. The currently accepted normal annual PSA increase is a maximum of 0.75 ng/ml; an increase above this value could indicate cancer and an increase below this value could point toward BPH or a normal prostate (see Fig. 3A). However, for PSA velocity to be a clinically useful tool, a man must have his blood tested at least three times over a period of at least two years. This gives a good overall picture of PSA production. PSA velocity is particularly useful in monitoring two types of patients:

- those whose PSA level is increasing rapidly but is still within the normal range (for example, if a 62-year-old man's PSA increases from 1.1 to 3.4 ng/ml in two years, his doctor may order a biopsy, even though the overall PSA level is still normal for his age); and

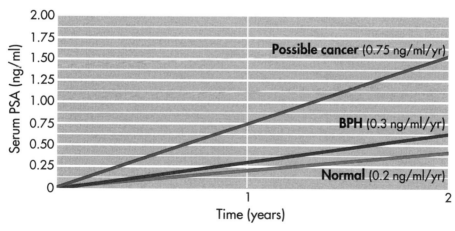

Fig. 3A — PSA Velocity

PSA velocity values (the change in the PSA level over time) for men with cancer, benign prostatic hyperplasia and a normal prostate.

- individuals with an elevated PSA level who have normal biopsy results (for example, if a patient has a PSA of 8.2 ng/ml but has a negative biopsy, the doctor can use PSA velocity to help determine whether a second biopsy will be necessary the following year. If the PSA level increases to 8.5 ng/ml, the doctor may not choose to biopsy again. If it rises to 9.6 ng/ml, however, a biopsy may be needed).

Studies have shown that PSA velocity is useful in reducing the number of unnecessary prostate biopsies. In men with BPH, for example, PSA velocity has reduced the number of biopsies from four in 10 to one in 10.

So even though the PSA blood test can detect prostate cancer while it is still curable and can reduce the number of needless biopsies in men with benign prostate enlargement, its use remains controversial for a variety of reasons.

Common arguments against using the PSA blood test:

- There has been no long-term, properly designed research study to show that early detection and subsequent treatment save lives.
- It may detect some cancers that are not "clinically significant," meaning that the tumor may be so small and grow so slowly that it might not be a threat to the man's life in the long run.
- It can give false-positive results, which means that some people may be led to believe they have prostate cancer when in fact they do not, which creates a lot of anxiety for the patient and unnecessary additional testing.
- Widespread use of the PSA test is expensive.

Common arguments in favor of PSA testing:

- There has been no long-term, properly designed research study to show that early detection and treatment do *not* save lives.
- Studies have shown that at least 85 percent of the prostate cancers being treated today are clinically significant, that is, potentially life-threatening.

- It can detect prostate cancers at a more localized, early stage while they are still curable. However, the PSA test must be used along with the DRE to ensure the most accurate results, just as breast self-exams should be used in tandem with mammography to detect breast cancer. Should we discourage women from having a mammogram because it may give a false-positive result? No. Therefore, should we discourage men from having a PSA test? Of course not.

- Long-term treatment is very expensive. You can spend some now to save a lot later, or you can save now and spend a lot more later.

So who is right and who is wrong? Future research will be the deciding factor. Two large national government studies are trying to help settle the controversy over PSA testing. One study is called PIVOT (Prostate Cancer Intervention vs. Observation Trial) and the other is called the PLCO (Prostate, Lung, Colon and Ovarian Cancer) Study.

The PIVOT study, conducted by the Department of Veterans Affairs and the National Cancer Institute, is comparing watchful waiting (no treatment) with radical prostatectomy (surgical removal of the prostate) among men with early, localized prostate cancer. It will involve 2,000 men up to age 75 and follow them for 12 years. This study will be especially useful in investigating quality-of-life issues related to treatment and non-treatment.

The PLCO study, directed by the National Cancer Institute, seeks to determine the impact of cancer screening on life expectancy. Men in this study will undergo PSA testing once a year for four years and then be followed without additional cancer screening for another 12 years. Men up to the age of 74 are being recruited. Because those diagnosed with prostate cancer during this study will be able to choose whatever treatment they want — or opt for no treatment at all — it will be difficult to tell whether PSA screening itself will make a difference in their long-term survival.

Whether you decide to have regular prostate exams (including the PSA test) or to undergo treatment if a cancer is found is a personal matter. Just because a prostate cancer is discovered does not automatically mean that you are headed for surgery. The choice of what to do is up to you, your family and your doctor, working together as a team. If the cancer is still confined to the prostate, you may opt for external-beam radiation, radiation seed implants, cryosurgery or radical prostatectomy, or you may choose the more conservative "watchful waiting" approach to see how fast the tumor grows before deciding if and when to proceed with treatment. The point is, the more objective information you have, the easier it is for you to make such a choice.

Patients should never be treated as if they are robots waiting to be programmed by their doctors. An objective and knowledgeable patient combined with an objective and knowledgeable doctor creates the strongest and most beneficial force in medicine. Once this force is created, the questions of "to test or not to test" and "to treat or not to treat" can be addressed individually and effectively.

Note:

Before the PSA test was developed, a test that measured levels of a substance called acid phosphatase was used to detect prostate cancer. While the PSA test is a superior method of cancer detection, some doctors still use the acid-phosphatase test along with the PSA test to help determine whether cancer has spread beyond the prostate.

FAST FACT

Five out of every 100 American men in their 60s will develop prostate cancer. The PSA test alone will detect cancer in three of these five men but will miss the cancer in the other two. An additional six men out of this group will receive a false-positive result from their PSA test, indicating the presence of cancer that isn't really there. The risk of missing cancer or falsely diagnosing the disease is part of the controversy over establishing massive PSA-based screening programs in the United States.

B

What factors could affect my PSA level?

Just because your PSA level is high or has increased does not necessarily mean you have cancer. Earlier in this chapter you learned about two common, noncancerous causes of PSA elevation: age-related enlargement of the prostate, or BPH; and prostatitis, or infection of the prostate gland. Below is a list of other conditions, medical procedures and medications that can trigger temporary changes in PSA:

Conditions

Acute urinary retention — This condition, in which urination becomes impossible, is often associated with severe enlargement of the prostate. Emergency medical intervention is required.

Ejaculation (orgasm) — Among men between 50-79 years of age, PSA levels rise significantly after ejaculation (see Fig. 3B). PSA levels increase up to 40 percent within an hour of ejaculation and return to normal within 48 hours. Therefore, men age 50 and older should refrain from sex for at least two days before undergoing a PSA test to ensure the most accurate results. Men in this age group can experience higher PSA levels after sex because the tissue barriers that keep the enzyme within the prostate, where it is manufactured, deteriorate with age; thus, older prostates can be more "leaky" than younger prostates. When a man ejaculates, the muscle of the prostate contracts and relaxes, which basically "massages" the gland. Among men in their 50s, 60s and 70s, this activity can allow PSA to escape more easily into the general circulation.

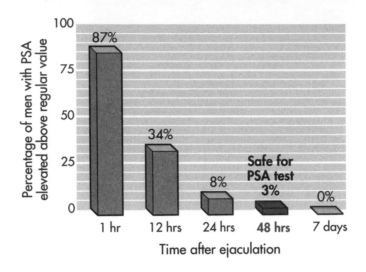

Fig. 3B — Effect of Ejaculation on PSA

After ejaculation, most men experience an increase in their PSA that can be large enough to falsely suggest the presence of cancer. However, after about 48 hours, the PSA level typically returns to normal.

Procedures

All of the following urological procedures cause a temporary elevation in the PSA level:

- Balloon dilation of the prostate
- High-intensity focused ultrasound (HIFU)
- Transrectal ultrasound (TRUS)-guided biopsy
- Transurethral incision of the prostate (TUIP)
- Transurethral microwave therapy (TUMT)
- Transurethral needle ablation (TUNA)
- Transurethral resection of the prostate (TURP)
- Visual laser ablation of the prostate (VLAP)

The following procedures DO NOT affect the PSA level:

- cystoscopy, flexible or rigid
- digital-rectal examination
- catheterization of the bladder
- the insertion of prostatic stents
- transrectal ultrasound, or TRUS, when performed without biopsy

After undergoing a prostate biopsy or any of the above treatments for benign prostatic enlargement, you should wait at least six weeks for the PSA level to return to baseline, or normal, before scheduling a cancer-screening test.

Medications

Finasteride (trade name Proscar) — This FDA-approved drug for benign prostatic hyperplasia helps shrink the prostate and may reduce symptoms associated with BPH. It also reduces the PSA level by 50 percent while you are taking it. If you are on Proscar and your doctor uses age-specific reference ranges, they would be cut in half. For example, if you are a 75 year old white male, your normal PSA reference range is 0-6.5 ng/ml; if you are taking Proscar, that range would drop to 0-3.25 ng/ml.

The following BPH medications DO NOT affect the PSA level:

- Doxazosin (trade name Cardura)
- Terazosin (trade name Hytrin)

(For a summary of all the factors that increase, decrease or have no effect on the PSA level, see Table 3B.)

Table 3B — The Various Procedures, Conditions and Medications That Can Affect a Man's PSA Test Result

May Increase Your PSA Result	May Decrease Your PSA Result	Does Not Influence Your PSA Result
Acute prostatitis	A medication for BPH called Finasteride (Proscar) from Merck decreases your PSA by half	Two medications for BPH called Doxazosin (Cardura) made by Pfizer and Terazosin (Hytrin) made by Abbott Labs
Acute urinary retention		
BPH procedures:	Too much bed rest	Catheterization of the bladder
Balloon dilation		
HIFU		DRE
TRUS		
TUIP		Flexible or rigid cystoscopy
TUMT		
TUNA		The insertion of prostatic stents
TURP		
VLAP		Transrectal ultrasound (TRUS) when done **WITHOUT** biopsy
Ejaculation (within 48 hours of your PSA test)		
Transrectal ultrasound (TRUS) when done **WITH** biopsy		

FAST FACT

The BPH medication finasteride (trade name Proscar) shows promise as a prostate-cancer prevention drug and may also be an effective treatment for male-pattern baldness. Results of clinical trials should be available within the next several years.

C

Are all PSA tests created equal?

Currently there are six FDA-approved PSA blood tests, or assays, on the market in the United States (see Table 3C); more than 30 are being used in Europe.

It is important to remember that not all of these tests are exactly the same. Therefore, PSA results can vary slightly, depending on which brand is used and which laboratory analyzes the test. The results of PSA tests performed on the same individual even hours or minutes apart can vary up to 8 percent, regardless of whether the same brand of test is used. These changes are not considered significant enough to be of concern, but to ensure the most consistent results, your annual PSA test should be processed by the same laboratory each time. If this isn't possible, then at least request that the same brand of test be used consistently.

Table 3C — Currently Available FDA-approved PSA Blood Tests

Blood Test	Manufacturer	Headquarters	Phone Number
PSA I & II	Chiron Diagnostics	Norwood, Mass.	(800) 255-3232
Immunolite	Diagnostic Products Corp.	Los Angeles, Calif.	(800) 372-1782
IMX	Abbott Laboratories	Abbott Park, Ill.	(800) 527-1869
Tandem-E	Hybritech Inc.	San Diego, Calif.	(800) 526-3821
Tandem-R	Hybritech Inc.	San Diego, Calif.	(800) 526-3821
Tosoh	Tosoh Medics Inc.	Foster City, Calif.	(800) 248-6764

One of the most exciting new developments concerning PSA testing is the discovery that the enzyme exists in the blood in a variety of molecular forms. This has led to the development of a new PSA test that increases the detection of the earliest, most curable prostate cancers while reducing the number of unnecessary prostate biopsies.

The new test, called the percent-free PSA test, is based on the recent discovery that PSA exists in the blood in both a "free" and "complexed" form. In the free state, PSA floats through the circulation by itself. In the complexed state, PSA hitches a ride on a protein called alpha1-antichymotrypsin as it journeys through the bloodstream. Together, the free and complexed forms make up the total PSA level that is measured by a standard PSA blood test.

Recently, researchers determined that men with benign prostatic enlargement have a greater amount of free PSA in their blood, while those with prostate cancer have more of the complexed variety (see Fig. 3C).

This new percent-free PSA test, not yet widely available, calculates the percentage of free PSA in the blood. This test is geared specifically for men who've been told that their PSA level is in the gray zone, between 3-10 ng/ml, to better determine whether they have a cancerous prostate or benign enlargement.

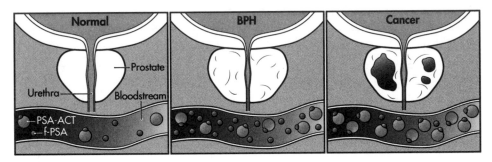

Fig. 3C — 'Free' and 'Complexed' PSA in the Bloodstream

"Free" and "complexed" molecular forms of PSA are deposited in the bloodstream in varying amounts, depending on the condition of the prostate. This is the basis of the new "percent-free PSA test." On the left is a normal prostate, which releases small amounts of both free (f-PSA) and complexed (PSA-ACT) PSA into the bloodstream. In the center is an enlarged, BPH-affected prostate, which typically releases higher amounts of free PSA than normal. On the right is a cancerous prostate, which usually releases more complexed PSA than normal.

In a recent study of more than 400 men, the new percent-free PSA test increased cancer detection by 44 percent among men with a total PSA level of 3-4 ng/ml. For those with a total reading between 4.1-10 ng/ml, this technique reduced the number of unnecessary (negative) biopsies by 15 percent. Traditionally, a prostate biopsy would be recommended for all men whose PSA falls within this latter range. Because the percent-free PSA test is a recent development in prostate-cancer detection, it is not yet FDA approved.

FAST FACT

MOLECULAR FORMS OF PSA

Forms of PSA	Description	Detected by the PSA Test
Free PSA (f-PSA)	PSA not attached to anything (5% to 40% of the PSA in the blood that is detected by a PSA test)	Yes
Complexed PSA (PSA-ACT)	PSA attached to a protein (65% to 90% of the PSA that is detected by a PSA test)	Yes
Total PSA (t-PSA)	All the PSA forms in the blood that are detected by a PSA test are made up of f-PSA and PSA-ACT	Yes
PSA-MG (also called "occult PSA" or "hidden PSA")	PSA completely surrounded by a protein so it is not detectable by the PSA test	No
PSA-AT	Only very small amount found in the blood	No
PSA-ITI	Only very small amount found in the blood	No
PSA-PCI	Only found in the semen	No

The ABCs of CHAPTER 3

A Quick Review

A

What is PSA? How do I understand my PSA test result? Why is there controversy about this test?

- PSA, or prostate-specific antigen, is an enzyme produced by the prostate. It is found in the bloodstream and the seminal fluid.

- Cancer isn't the only factor that causes the PSA level to increase. For this reason, PSA is not a perfect test for prostate cancer, but it is the most clinically useful tumor marker available today.

- The normal PSA range is 0-4 ng/ml. A reading from 4-10 ng/ml is less conclusive; a reading above 10 ng/ml is a likely indication of cancer, but only a prostate biopsy can tell for sure. However, the use of age-specific reference ranges increases cancer detection in younger men and decreases prostate biopsies in older men.

- PSA velocity (measuring the increase in PSA level over time) is a clinically useful cancer-detection tool, but only if the PSA is measured for two consecutive years to obtain an accurate picture of PSA production. The upper limit of normal for an annual PSA increase is 0.75 ng/ml.

B

What factors can affect my PSA level?

- Conditions that can cause PSA to rise include age, ejaculation, infection and urinary retention.

- Procedures that can cause a temporary spike in PSA include transrectal ultrasound-guided prostate biopsy and a wide variety of treatments for benign prostatic enlargement.

- The FDA-approved BPH medication finasteride (trade name Proscar) reduces the PSA level by 50 percent while a person is taking it. If you are on Proscar, your doctor should take this into account when interpreting your PSA result, reducing your age-specific reference range by half.

C

Are all PSA tests created equal?

- There are currently six FDA-approved PSA tests on the market in the United States, and more than 30 in Europe. While the tests are very similar, PSA results can vary up to 8 percent, depending on which brand is used and which laboratory processes the test. Ideally, your tests should be sent to the same lab each time, or your doctor should consistently use the same brand of test.

- A recent discovery that PSA exists in a number of molecular forms has led to a newer, more accurate cancer-screening tool called the "percent-free" PSA test.

- Not yet widely available, this test detects the amount of free PSA in the blood. Knowing this level will allow doctors to better determine whether a patient with slightly elevated PSA — in the gray zone — indeed may have prostate cancer. Researchers hope this test will significantly increase the detection of early, curable prostate tumors and decrease the performance of unnecessary prostate biopsies.

Medical References

Title: **"Free, complexed and total serum prostate-specific antigen: the establishment of appropriate reference ranges for their concentrations and ratios"**
Authors: Oesterling, J.E.; Jacobsen, S.J.; Klee, G.G.; et al
Journal: *Journal of Urology*
Volume: 154 (3)
Pages: 1090-1095
Date: September 1995

Title: **"Evaluation of percentage of free serum prostate-specific antigen to improve specificity of prostate cancer screening"**
Authors: Catalona, W.J.; Smith, D.S.; Wolfert, R.L.; et al
Journal: *Journal of the American Medical Association (JAMA)*
Volume: 274 (15)
Pages: 1214-1220
Date: Oct. 18, 1995

Title: **"The clinical usefulness of prostate-specific antigen: update 1994"**
Authors: Partin, A.W.; and Oesterling, J.E.
Journal: *Journal of Urology*
Volume: 152 (5 pt 1)
Pages: 1358-1368
Date: November 1994

Title: **"Serum prostate-specific antigen in a community-based population of healthy men. Establishment of age-specific reference ranges."**
Authors: Oesterling, J.E.; Jacobsen, S.J.; Chute, C.G.; et al
Journal: *New England Journal of Medicine*
Volume: 270 (7)
Pages: 860-864
Date: Aug. 18, 1993

Title: **"Measurement of prostate-specific antigen in serum as a screening test for prostate cancer"**
Authors: Catalona, W.J.; Smith, D.S.: Ratliff, T.L.; et al
Journal: *New England Journal of Medicine*
Volume: 324 (17)
Pages: 1156-1161
Date: April 25, 1991

4

Things You Should Know Even if You Don't Have Prostate Cancer

A

So, my prostate is normal.
Does this mean I'm off the hook?

B

What is benign prostatic hyperplasia,
or BPH?

C

What is prostatitis?

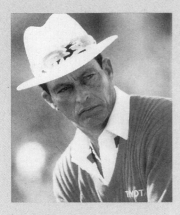

Chi Chi Rodriguez
Senior professional golfer

In the same amount of time it takes to drive to your local golf course or just walk up the 18th fairway, your life can be saved by a prostate checkup. A prostate checkup is simple, fast and only needs to be done once a year. Prostate cancer is now the leading cause of cancer in men, but if caught early, it is curable, and that is what we need to remember. Fortunately, I do not have prostate cancer, but I never miss my yearly exam.

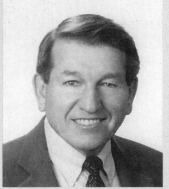

Johnny Unitas
Hall of Fame quarterback

I used to be a very sound sleeper. But in the summer of '95 I started getting up during the night to go to the bathroom sometimes two, three and four times a night. It started to really bother me and my wife, because it would keep her awake. We talked about it and agreed that I should go to see my doctor.

I went to my doctor and he told me I do not have cancer, which was a great relief to me and my wife. But I found out I do have benign prostate enlargement. We talked about my symptoms and together we decided to just watch and wait. Now, I keep an eye on my symptoms and I see my doctor every three months.

The most important point is that I know what is going on, and so does my doctor. If it gets worse we know we can decide on the best course of action. ... And it all started with me talking to the doctor.

A
So, my prostate is normal.
Does this mean I'm off the hook?

Great news — you had a prostate exam and were told that your PSA and DRE results were normal — you don't have prostate cancer! However, you are still at risk of getting prostate cancer, so you should return every year for a prostate checkup (see Fig. 4A). Annual exams give you the best chance of diagnosing cancer early so that you can have the widest range of treatment options and the best chance of survival.

And even if your prostate is normal, you are still at risk of developing other prostate diseases such as noncancerous prostate enlargement (more commonly known as BPH, or benign prostatic hyperplasia) or prostatitis, a condition in which the prostate becomes inflamed and/or infected (see Table 4A).

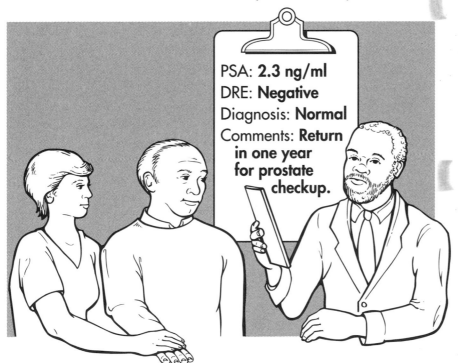

Fig. 4A — Annual Prostate Evaluation

Even if your prostate exam is normal, you still need to return each year for a checkup.

Table 4A — Diseases of the Prostate

Disease	Can It Increase Your PSA Level?	Can It Be Felt on DRE?	Can It Be Detected by Ultrasound?
BPH	Yes	Yes	Yes
Prostate Cancer	Yes	Yes	Yes
Prostatitis (*Acute bacterial, chronic bacterial, nonbacterial or prostatodynia*)	Yes	Yes*	Yes**

*If the condition is acute

**If it has progressed to a prostatic abscess.

FAST FACT

About seven out of every 10 men (70 percent) report no symptoms at the time of prostate-cancer diagnosis, which is another compelling reason for getting your prostate examined regularly.

B

What is benign prostatic hyperplasia, or BPH?

Benign prostatic hyperplasia (also called prostatism) is a non-cancerous condition in which the number of prostate cells increases, causing the gland to enlarge. BPH should not be confused with a condition called benign prostatic hypertrophy, in which the actual size of the prostate cells increases.

The word "benign" in BPH means the condition has no relation to cancer; BPH and cancer are separate conditions that have no relation to each other.

So why is BPH a problem if it is not cancerous? Because an enlarged prostate can put pressure on the urethra, squeezing the sides of the urinary tract together like a pinched straw, resulting in urinary problems. The area of the prostate affected by BPH is called the "transition" zone (see Fig. 4B).

Nearly all men will develop BPH if they live long enough; it is more commonplace than the common cold among older men. Half of those who get BPH will develop symptoms ranging from difficult urination and incontinence to infections of the urinary tract and bladder. A quarter to a third of these men will experience symptoms severe enough to require treatment. One in three to four men (25 percent to 33 percent) above age 50 will need some type of therapy to relieve the problems caused by BPH. Transurethral resection of the prostate (TURP), the traditional treatment for BPH, is the most common operation in men over age 55 in the United States, with some 250,000 procedures performed annually.

Age-related incidence of BPH

Age 40 to 50 — one in six men (17%)
Age 50 to 60 — one in four men (25%)
Age 60 and above — one in two men (50%)
Age 80 and above — one in 1.2 men (about 80%)

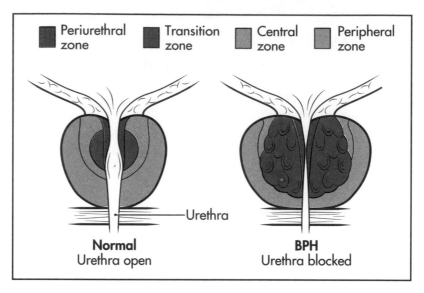

Periurethral zone   Transition zone   Central zone   Peripheral zone

Urethra

Normal
Urethra open

BPH
Urethra blocked

Fig. 4B — Normal vs. Enlarged Prostate

An enlarged prostate can put pressure on the urethra, squeezing the sides of the urinary tract together like a pinched straw, resulting in urinary problems.

BPH can begin when a man is in his 20s, but at this point the changes are still microscopic, undetectable by an exam. As one gets older, "microscopic" BPH can turn into "macroscopic" BPH, which means that enlargement of the prostate can be felt during a rectal exam but the changes aren't severe enough to cause symptoms. Macroscopic BPH eventually may develop into "clinical" BPH, in which a man experiences symptoms such as difficult urination.

The most common symptoms of urinary difficulty include:
- weak urine flow, or dribbling;
- having to push or strain to begin urine flow;
- urine flow that stops or starts a number of times before the bladder is empty;
- inability to empty the bladder completely;
- inability to urinate at all;

- difficulty holding one's urine or needing to urinate immediately;
- interrupted sleep due to the constant need to urinate at night; and
- wetting or staining the underwear.

If you are having any of the above problems, you should see your doctor.

It is important to remember that urinary problems do not automatically indicate the presence of BPH. They could also be a symptom of:

- a bladder stone;
- a bladder infection;
- a prostate infection;
- bladder complications caused by a neurological problem;
- narrowing of the urethra (also called a stricture);
- prostate cancer; or
- urinary problems caused by medication.

Because urinary difficulty can signify a wide variety of conditions, it is important to see your doctor at the first sign of trouble.

When you go to the doctor, you likely will be asked to fill out a questionnaire developed by the American Urological Association, or AUA, that asks about your ability to urinate in the past month. The doctor will use your answers to develop a "symptom score" to determine the severity of your problem (see Table 4B-1).

If you score 0-7, that means your symptoms are mild. A score of 8-18 indicates your problem is moderate and a result of 19-35 means your symptoms are severe. Your treatment options will be based on your overall symptom score.

Table 4B-1 — AUA Symptom Score for BPH

Questions

1. During the past month or so, how often have you had a sensation of not emptying your bladder completely after you finished urinating?

2. During the past month or so, how often have you had to urinate again less than two hours after you finished urinating?

3. During the past month or so, how often have you found you stopped and started again several times when you urinated?

4. During the past month or so, how often have you found it difficult to postpone urination?

5. During the past month or so, how often have you had a weak urinary stream?

6. During the past month or so, how often have you had to push or strain to begin urination?

7. During the last month, how many times did you most typically get up to urinate from the time you went to bed at night until the time you woke up in the morning?

Scoring for Possible Answers to Questions 1-6:

0 = Not at all
1 = Less than one time in five
2 = Less than half the time
3 = About half the time
4 = More than half the time
5 = Almost always

Scoring for Possible Answers to Question 7:

0 = Not at all
1 = one time
2 = two times
3 = three times
4 = four times
5 = ≥ five times

Symptom Score (Sum of the Answers)

0-7: mild BPH; 8-18: moderate BPH; 19-35: severe BPH

Source: *Journal of Urology*, Volume 148, Page 1557, November 1992.

In addition to the AUA questionnaire you can expect to undergo some tests, including:

- **a digital-rectal exam, or DRE,** to help determine the size of the prostate and rule out prostate cancer as a cause of the symptoms. (A normal prostate is usually no larger than a golf ball, while a prostate affected by BPH can become as large as a baseball);

- **a urine test (also called a urinalysis)** to detect any infections or other conditions that could produce symptoms similar to BPH;

- **a PSA (prostate-specific antigen)** blood test to check the prostate for the possibility of cancer. Up to half of all men with BPH experience a moderate rise in PSA, while 10 percent of men with BPH have a PSA level of 10 ng/ml or higher (PSA increase is roughly equal to the degree of prostate enlargement); and

- **a serum creatinine blood test** to measure kidney function, since up to 10 percent of men with BPH have some degree of kidney problems.

Depending on what the above tests show, your doctor may ask you to undergo the following four additional tests:

- **a peak urinary-flow test** to determine the strength of your urine stream and how much urine you can void at one time. The test is simple; after your bladder is full, you are asked to urinate into a funnel-like device that measures the strength (milliliters/second) and amount of urine (milliliters) delivered. A flow rate of greater than 15 ml/sec may indicate mild BPH or a normal condition. A flow rate of 10-15 ml/sec may indicate moderate BPH, and a flow rate of less than 10 ml/sec may indicate severe BPH (it also could mean that you simply have a weak bladder);

- **a residual urine-volume test** to see whether your bladder empties completely after urinating. This is also called a post-void residual volume, or PVR, test. Residual urine volume can be measured in two ways: by placing a small catheter into the penis and up into the bladder, or by placing an ultrasound transducer on top of your lower abdomen. The ultrasound method (also called transabdominal ultrasound) is more common but less accurate than the catheter method. Before determining treatment, several residual urine-volume tests may be performed, as the results can vary from time to time. A consistent residual volume above 100 ml is significant and warrants further evaluation;

- **a cystoscopic evaluation** to see whether the urinary problems are caused by an enlarged prostate and to see whether the bladder has been affected by the enlarging prostate. In cystoscopic evaluation, the doctor inserts a tiny illuminated scope (about the size of a pencil) into the penis to view the bladder and prostate. The procedure takes about five minutes and causes little or no discomfort, especially when performed with a flexible scope; and

- **a urine pressure/flow test** to measure bladder pressure during urination. This test, which involves the use of a thin catheter placed through the urethra, is used in patients whose previous test results have been inconclusive. This test is valuable in determining whether urinary problems are from an enlarged prostate or a weak bladder.

If you are diagnosed with BPH, you should know that within five years, the chances of your condition getting better are 15 percent, the chances of it staying the same are 30 percent and the odds of it getting worse are 55 percent.

If you decide to go the treatment route, the good news is that there are many good options; the bad news is that the most effective treatments are usually the most invasive and carry the greatest risk of complications.

Nonmedical treatment options for BPH

Watchful waiting — This means opting to carefully monitor the condition instead of pursuing immediate treatment. This is usually the preferred option for those whose BPH symptoms are mild or not bothersome. Watchful waiting is a very active process between the patient and his doctor, requiring men to see their doctor every six to 12 months for evaluation. If the condition worsens, a variety of medications and treatments, both minimally invasive and surgical, are available. In the meantime, it is important to limit certain medications that can make the condition worse, such as decongestants. It also helps not to drink alcohol or coffee after dinner or any other fluids right before bedtime.

Medical treatments for BPH

There are two types of drugs used in the treatment of BPH: five-alpha reductase inhibitors, which shrink the prostate; and alpha blockers, which relax the prostatic tissue (see Table 4B-2). Within these two classes of drugs there are currently three FDA-approved BPH medications on the market, all of which can be effective as long as they are taken.

Five-alpha reductase inhibitors — This type of drug blocks the action of the enzyme called five-alpha reductase, which converts testosterone into the powerful male hormone dihydrotestosterone (DHT). Inhibiting this enzyme causes the prostate to shrink, which then decreases the amount of urinary obstruction. This type of drug decreases the size of the prostate by 30 percent in two-thirds of those who take it. However, it takes about three to six months before symptoms start to improve.

The one FDA-approved five-alpha reductase inhibitor is called Proscar (finasteride), and it is made by Merck & Co. Inc. It is a pill that needs to be taken every day. In addition to decreasing the size of prostate, Proscar also may be effective in preventing prostate

Table 4B-2 — **Report Card:** *BPH Medications*

	Proscar (Five-alpha reductase inhibitor)	Cardura, Hytrin (Alpha blockers)
✔ **Effectiveness**		
Chance of symptom improvement	54-78%	59-86%
Percentage of symptom improvement	31%	51%
Five-year failure rate	10-27%	13-39%
Time it takes to work	3-6 months	2-6 weeks
✔ **Side effects**		
Impotence risk	3-5%	2%
Risk of decreased sex drive	3-4%	< 1%
Risk of retrograde ejaculation	< 1%	4-11%
Risk of drowsiness and headaches	< 1%	10-15%
Risk of dizziness and low blood pressure	< 1%	2-5%
✔ **Total average cost per year**	$700-$1,400	$700-$1,400

Drug treatment for BPH should NOT be considered for patients with:

- acute urinary retention (total blockage of urination);
- bladder stones or diverticula (outpouching of the bladder);
- kidney problems;
- residual urine volume greater than 300 ml;
- prostate cancer;
- recurrent blood in the urine; or
- recurrent urinary-tract infections caused by BPH.

FAST FACT

An interesting note about five-alpha reductase inhibitors and alpha blockers is that during clinical trials to determine their effectiveness, men receiving placebos (inactive sugar pills) had a 30-percent improvement in their ability to urinate.

cancer. Its potential in this area is currently being evaluated in the Prostate Cancer Prevention Trial, one of the largest clinical trials in U.S. history. Results of the study will be available in several years. Proscar also is being tested as a promising treatment for male-pattern baldness; results regarding this treatment also should be available in several years.

Alpha blockers — Alpha blockers work by relaxing the prostate, which decreases the amount of pressure on the urethra and thus relieves urinary obstruction. Alpha blockers are pills that need to be taken once a day, and they require at least two to six weeks to start working noticeably. If symptoms don't improve within two to four months, another type of treatment should be considered.

The FDA-approved alpha blockers are Cardura (doxazosin), made by Pfizer Pharmaceuticals; and Hytrin (terazosin), made by Abbott Laboratories. Another alpha blocker called Tamsulosin, made by Yamanouchi, soon may be approved by the FDA. Initial results show it to be similar to the other alpha blockers in effectiveness and complication risk.

Minimally invasive treatments for BPH

There are several minimally invasive treatments for BPH that use a variety of tools, from lasers to electrical rollerballs, to zap over-grown prostate tissue and restore urine flow.

Transurethral needle ablation, or TUNA — This is a catheter-based procedure that recently gained FDA approval. It relies on low-level radiofrequency, or RF, energy to selectively target and shrink prostate tissue. Performed under local anesthesia, the urologist uses a fiber-optic image to direct a special catheter into the portion of the urethra that passes through the prostate gland. Two needles, covered by protective shields, are deployed from the catheter into the prostate. The shields are retracted to expose the needles, which then deliver the RF energy to specific locations in the gland. Because the needles are covered, the urethra itself is protected; only the prostate tissue is destroyed. Based on preliminary results, symptom improvement with TUNA is similar to that of TURP. Very little bleeding occurs with TUNA. Approximately 40 percent of patients require a catheter for a certain amount of time after the procedure.

A recent multicenter study that compared TUNA to traditional surgical treatment found that side effects such as impotence, incontinence and retrograde ejaculation can be virtually avoided with this technique.

Transurethral incision of the prostate, or TUIP — This minimally invasive outpatient or overnight procedure, performed under either local or general anesthesia, involves making an incision from the bladder neck down through the portion of the prostate tissue that covers the urethra. This helps to open up the bladder neck and urethra and relieve the obstruction (see Table 4B-3).

Table 4B-3 — **Report Card:** *TUIP*

✔ **Effectiveness**

Chance of symptom improvement	90 %
Amount of reduction in symptom score	73 %
Average peak urine flow increase	8-15 ml/sec
Chance of needing more treatment within eight years	20 %

✔ **Side effects**

Overall complication risk	14 %
Impotence risk	2-4 %
Risk of retrograde ejaculation	15-20 %
Need for additional surgery to correct complications of TUIP	3 %
Risk of blood transfusion	2 %
Risk of incontinence	< 1 %
Risk of death	< 1 %

✔ **Total average cost** | $2,000-$4,000 |

Transurethral microwave thermotherapy, or TUMT — This procedure, performed in a single session without anesthesia, involves delivering microwave energy to the prostate through a wire-covered catheter that is kept cool on the outside to protect the urethra. The energy is delivered from a device called a Prostatron machine. Approximately one in four patients experiences temporary urine retention and requires an indwelling catheter for several days after the procedure.

Visual laser ablation of the prostate, or VLAP — This type of treatment involves sending laser energy through a catheter inside the urethra to "cook" obstructing prostate tissue. The dead tissue is then absorbed by the body or sloughed away during urination. Because the urethra is exposed to laser energy, this outpatient technique requires general or spinal anesthesia and temporary catheterization to allow the urethra to heal.

Because blood loss is kept to a minimum, VLAP probably is ideal for men receiving anticoagulation therapy. For these individuals, it is not necessary to stop using blood-thinning drugs such as heparin, warfarin or nonsteroidal anti-inflammatory medications before the procedure. However, patients may experience pain and problems passing urine immediately after the procedure. Therefore, all patients need a catheter for several days after VLAP. Long-term studies are needed before VLAP can be given a complete report card.

Electrovaporization of the prostate, or EVP — This is a 35- to 50-minute procedure in which electrical currents are used to vaporize obstructing prostate tissue. Currents are delivered through a rollerball electrode inside the urethra. The main advantages of EVP, which is performed under general or spinal anesthesia, are that there's no bleeding and, for many, no catheterization or overnight hospital stay is necessary. Long-term studies are needed before a full report card can be given. However, in the short-term EVP is similar to transurethral resection of the prostate, the surgical gold standard, with regard to average procedure time, symptom improvement and cost. (For more about this procedure, see below.)

Surgical treatments for BPH

Transurethral resection of the prostate, or TURP, and open prostatectomy are two separate surgical procedures for the treatment of BPH, but both have much in common (see Table 4B-4). Both result in the greatest improvement of symptoms and urinary flow compared to the other BPH treatments, and both allow the prostate tissue that is removed to be examined for cancer, if necessary.

TURP involves passing a heated wire loop through the urethra, which is used to peel away obstructing prostatic tissue and thus relieve pressure on the urethra. The irritation caused by the cutting wire can lead to a variety of postsurgical complications, from impotence to retrograde ejaculation (when the ejaculate produced during an orgasm backs up into the bladder instead of exiting the body through the penis).

There are two types of open prostatectomy:

- **retropubic prostatectomy**, in which an incision is made in the lower abdomen and the prostate capsule is cut; and

- **suprapubic (transvesical) prostatectomy**, in which the surgeon accesses the prostate by cutting through the bladder.

Open prostatectomy is more invasive, requires a longer hospital stay and carries a higher risk of postoperative complications than TURP. Therefore, the majority of doctors and patients today prefer TURP over open prostatectomy, except in cases where the prostate has become very large (more than 80-100 grams).

Table 4B-4 — **Report Card:** *TURP vs. Open Prostatectomy*

	TURP	Open Prostatectomy
✔ **Effectiveness**		
Chance of symptom improvement	75-96%	94-100%
Symptom-score improvement	85%	90%
Improvement in urinary-flow rate	8-18 ml/sec	8-23 ml/sec
Need for more treatment eight years after initial surgery	16-20%	10%
✔ **Side effects**		
Complication risk	16%	22%
Risk of retrograde ejaculation	80-90%	85-95%
Risk of blood transfusion	5-7%	30%
Risk of impotence	3-5%	7-10%
Risk of incontinence	<1%	<1%
Risk of death	1%	2%
✔ **Total average cost**	$4,000-$6,000	$10,000-$15,00

Experimental BPH treatments (not FDA approved)

Transrectal high-intensity focused ultrasound, or HIFU — A procedure in which an ultrasound probe is placed in the rectum, which heats the prostate (up to 100 degrees Celsius) with ultrasound waves without hurting the rectal wall. The heat destroys excess prostate tissue, which decreases BPH symptoms and increases urinary flow. HIFU is a promising treatment, but very little information exists currently on its effectiveness, safety and long-term results.

Prostatic stents — Stents are tiny springs used to keep the urethra open so urine can flow. Temporary and permanent stents have been used to enlarge the portion of the urethra that runs through the prostate. However, the prostate tissue can grow between the wire coils and the stent itself can become covered with calcium salts, causing pain and irritation. Therefore, the individuals who best qualify for stents are those with urinary retention who are not candidates for surgery.

Balloon dilation — This treatment received some attention in the early 90s, but the overall results have been disappointing. The procedure involves inserting a deflated balloon into the urethra through a catheter. When the balloon reaches the portion of the catheter that runs through the prostate, it is inflated to widen the urethra and is then removed. Most long-term studies have shown very little improvement in urinary symptoms, therefore, the use of this treatment has become almost nonexistent.

FAST FACT

The most common surgery in the world is for cataracts. The second most common surgery in the world is for BPH.

C
What is prostatitis?

Any medical term with the suffix "-itis" on the end refers to inflammation or swelling. For example, tonsillitis is an inflammation or swelling of the tonsils, usually caused by an infection. So, prostatitis is an inflammation or swelling of the prostate, which can be caused by a variety of factors. Having prostatitis does not affect your risk of getting prostate cancer.

There are four types of prostatitis (see Fig. 4C, Table 4C):

Acute bacterial — a sudden bacterial infection characterized by fever and chills, pain in the lower back and in the area between the rectum and testicles, painful urination and the urgent need to urinate. Treatment: six to 12 weeks of antibiotics.

Chronic bacterial — a long-lasting or recurring bacterial infection characterized by painful urination, pain in the pelvis and genital area, frequent, difficult urination and the urgent need to urinate. Treatment: three to six weeks of antibiotics.

Nonbacterial — inflammation of unknown origin characterized by painful urination. Treatment: frequent hot baths and over-the-counter anti-inflammatory drugs or muscle relaxants such as alpha blockers used to treat BPH, such as Hytrin and Cardura. A change in diet also may help, such as a decrease in spicy foods, alcohol and caffeine.

Prostatodynia — painful inflammation caused by muscle spasms, characterized by painful urination. Treatment is the same as for nonbacterial prostatitis, above.

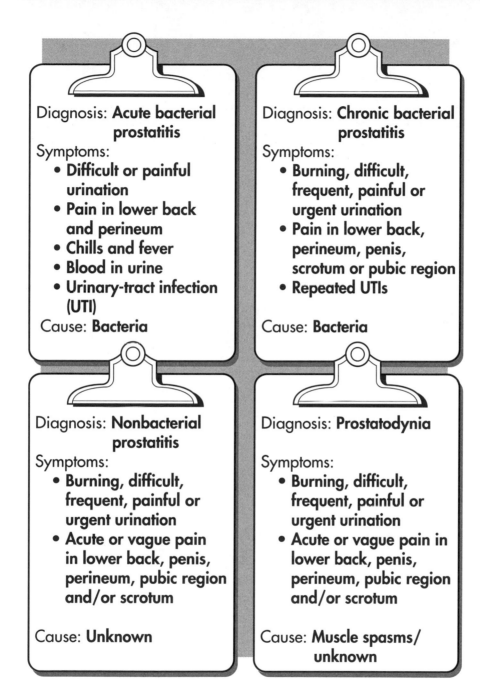

Diagnosis: **Acute bacterial prostatitis**

Symptoms:
- **Difficult or painful urination**
- **Pain in lower back and perineum**
- **Chills and fever**
- **Blood in urine**
- **Urinary-tract infection (UTI)**

Cause: **Bacteria**

Diagnosis: **Chronic bacterial prostatitis**

Symptoms:
- **Burning, difficult, frequent, painful or urgent urination**
- **Pain in lower back, perineum, penis, scrotum or pubic region**
- **Repeated UTIs**

Cause: **Bacteria**

Diagnosis: **Nonbacterial prostatitis**

Symptoms:
- **Burning, difficult, frequent, painful or urgent urination**
- **Acute or vague pain in lower back, penis, perineum, pubic region and/or scrotum**

Cause: **Unknown**

Diagnosis: **Prostatodynia**

Symptoms:
- **Burning, difficult, frequent, painful or urgent urination**
- **Acute or vague pain in lower back, penis, perineum, pubic region and/or scrotum**

Cause: **Muscle spasms/ unknown**

Fig. 4C — The Four Types of Prostatitis

The four varieties of prostatitis share many features, which can make diagnosis difficult when based on symptoms alone.

Table 4C — Clinical Characteristics of Prostatitis

What are the different types of prostatitis?	In what percentage of prostatitis patients does this type occur?	Is the prostate abnormal in rectal exam?	Is there a higher than normal white blood count in prostatic secretions?	Can it be treated with antibiotics?	Does it decrease the urinary flow rate?
Acute bacterial	1-5 %	Yes	Yes	Yes	Yes
Chronic bacterial	1-5 %	Maybe	Yes	Yes	Maybe
Nonbacterial	64 %	Maybe	Yes	No	Maybe
Prostatodynia	31 %	No	No	No	Yes

Note:

Bacterial prostatitis is also sometimes called infectious prostatitis. However, prostatitis is NOT infectious; it cannot be passed from one person to another through any type of contact, including sexual intercourse. This is true for all types of prostatitis, as well as for BPH and prostate cancer — none of these disorders is contagious. However, with unprotected anal sex, bacteria from the rectum can enter the urethra and find their way to the prostate, thus causing the prostate to become infected.

FAST FACT

Two percent of all doctor visits for urinary and genital problems are due to prostatitis.

The ABCs of CHAPTER 4

A Quick Review

A

So, my prostate is normal. Does this mean I'm off the hook?

- Most men will leave their annual prostate checkup with a clean bill of health; if your PSA and DRE results are normal, there is a 91 percent to 95 percent chance that you do not have cancer.

- Even if your results are normal, you still need to come back once a year for a PSA checkup.

- The other common prostate diseases that can be diagnosed during the annual exam are benign prostatic hyperplasia (enlargement) and prostatitis (infection/inflammation).

B

What is benign prostatic hyperplasia, or BPH?

- BPH (also called prostattism) is the noncancerous enlargement of the prostate gland. The condition is almost as commonplace as the common cold in men over the age of 50.

- BPH causes the urethra to narrow, which can result in urinary problems.

- The more invasive the treatment for BPH, the more effective the treatment.

  The two types of BPH medications are five-alpha reductase inhibitors, which shrink the prostate; and alpha blockers, which relax the prostate.

  Minimally invasive treatments for BPH include transurethral needle ablation (TUNA), transurethral incision of the prostate (TUIP), transurethral microwave thermotherapy

(TUMT), visual laser ablation of the prostate (VLAP) and electrovaporization of the prostate (EVP).

Surgical treatment options for BPH are transurethral resection of the prostate (TURP) and open prostatectomy.

Investigational (non-FDA-approved) treatments for BPH include transrectal high-intensity focused ultrasound (HIFU), prostatic stents and balloon dilation.

- The two bacterial types of prostatitis can be treated with antibiotics.

  The other two types can be treated with muscle-relaxing drugs, hot baths, pain medications and dietary changes.

- Prostatitis **CANNOT** be transmitted from person to person.

C

What is prostatitis?

- Prostatitis is inflammation and/or infection of the prostate. There are four types of prostatitis: acute and chronic bacterial, non-bacterial and prostatodynia. It is not easy to diagnose the specific type of prostatitis because each share many common symptoms.

Medical References

Title: **"Benign prostatic hyperplasia. Medical and minimally invasive treatment options."**
Author: Oesterling, J.E.
Journal: *New England Journal of Medicine*
Volume: 332 (2)
Pages: 99-109
Date: Jan. 12, 1995

Title: **"A comparison of transurethral surgery with watchful waiting for moderate symptoms of benign prostatic hyperplasia. The Veterans Affairs Study Group on Transurethral Resection of the Prostate."**
Authors: Wasson, J.H.; Reda, D.J.; Bruskewitz, R.C.; et al
Journal: *New England Journal of Medicine*
Volume: 332 (2)
Pages: 75-79
Date: Jan. 12, 1995

Title: **"Prostatic fluid inflammation in prostatitis."**
Authors: Wright, E.T.; Chmiel, J.S.; Grayhack, J.T.; et al
Journal: *Journal of Urology*
Volume: 152 (6 pt 2)
Pages: 2300-2303
Date: December 1994

Title: **"Benign prostatic hyperplasia: its natural history, epidemiologic characteristics, and surgical treatment."**
Author: Oesterling, J.E.
Journal: *Archives of Family Medicine*
Volume: 1
Pages: 257-266
Date: November 1992

Title: **"The American Urological Association symptom index for benign prostatic hyperplasia. The Measurement Committee of the American Urological Association."**
Authors: Barry, M.J.; Fowler, F.J.; O'Leary, M.P.; et al
Journal: *Journal of Urology*
Volume: 148 (5)
Pages: 1549-1557, 1564 (discussion)
Date: November 1992

Notes _____

_____

_____

_____

_____

_____

_____

_____

_____

_____

_____

_____

_____

_____

_____

_____

_____

_____

_____

_____

_____

5

The Biopsy is Positive:
It's Prostate Cancer

A

What is the Gleason
grading system?

B

What are the ABCD and
TNM staging systems?

C

What tests might I need to see
whether my cancer has spread?

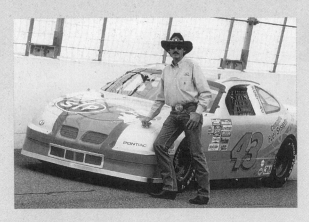

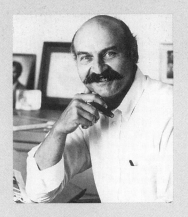

Richard Petty
Champion stock-car racer

When I was told I had prostate cancer, the very first question I asked my doctor, without hesitation, was, "Can we get it out tomorrow?" I have always been the type of person who believes when something is broken it should be fixed. This is how I felt that day — if something is out of order with my body, it should be fixed.

As owner of Petty Enterprises, a company that builds car No. 43 and races in the Winston Cup Division, it is essential that we build and maintain the highest-quality race car. While preparing a race car we use a checklist before each race to detect any hidden problems and make sure the car keeps running smoothly. A person should treat their body in the same fashion. If I had not had my yearly prostate checkup, the doctor may not have found the prostate cancer in time and I might have crossed the finish line way too soon.

Always have your yearly checkup, which should include a digital-rectal exam and PSA test. This could be your most important road test.

Jim Berry
Cartoonist ('Berry's World')

When the doctor said, "I'm sorry, Mr. Berry, but you have a malignant growth in your prostate," I said, "Now, wait a minute. I'm too young for this. This is the kind of thing that happens to other people." It really hit me. I was only 58, I had no symptoms, and my rectal exam had been normal. It was the PSA blood test that found my cancer, which, thankfully, was still confined to the prostate. If I hadn't had the PSA test, my cancer may not have been discovered in time to have been successfully treated.

My message to any man who is procrastinating about seeing his doctor and getting a regular physical is: DON'T. You should go, because even if you're diagnosed with prostate cancer, there is technology today that can help you lead a normal life after treatment.

Berry's World

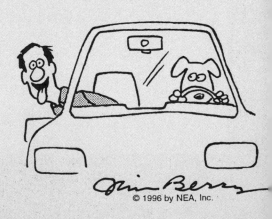

A

What is the Gleason grading system?

So your doctor has found cancer in your biopsy. But because not all prostate cancers look or act the same, it is time to "grade" your cancer to determine how aggressive, or fast-growing, it is.

The grading technique used most often is called the Gleason grading system. This requires a pathologist to examine tissue specimens from two of the most representative areas of the tumor. After studying these tissue samples under a microscope, the pathologist assigns each a grade between 1 and 5. (Grade 1 means the cancer is not very aggressive and is unlikely to spread quickly, while grade 5 means it is very likely to grow fast.) The two grades that occur most often in the samples are then recorded (see Fig. 5A).

Then, the pathologist adds the two grades together to arrive at an overall score of between 2 and 10. A score of 2-4 means the cancer is growing slowly, while a score of 8-10 means the cancer is growing quickly. So, the lower the Gleason score, the less aggressive the cancer. A score somewhere in the middle, between 5-7, can be either slow- or fast-growing. This is the "gray area" of prostate-cancer grading.

It is interesting that some high-grade prostate cancers with overall scores between 8-10 (also called "non-differentiated" or "poorly differentiated" tumors) do not increase a man's PSA level dramatically. This is probably due to the fact that those cancers look and act very differently from normal prostate tissue. Therefore, they do not release as much PSA. On the other hand, some low-grade cancers with scores between 2-4 (also known as "differentiated" or "well-differentiated" tumors) dramatically increase a man's PSA level. This is probably due to the fact that these cancers look and act similarly to normal prostate tissue, therefore they release PSA. Some moderate-grade cancers with scores between 5-7 can produce significant quantities of PSA, while others do not change a man's PSA level at all, so this is also why we call this range the "gray zone" (see Table 5A).

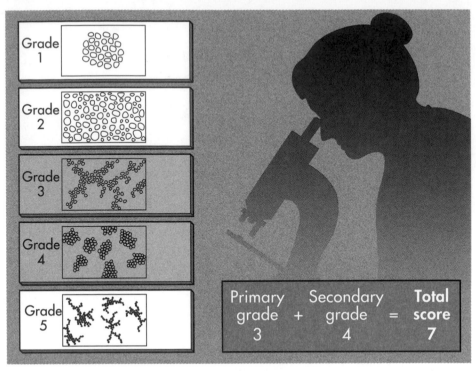

Fig. 5A — The Gleason Grading System

A pathologist (also called a uro-pathologist) studies your prostate cancer on a series of slides under a microscope. Keep in mind that a cancer specimen does not look the same throughout; the size and shape of cancer cells vary from one part of the tumor to another. The type of cancer cell that takes up the largest area on your slides is what determines your cancer's primary grade, which is ranked from 1 to 5. The type of cancer cell that takes up the second largest area on the slides determines your cancer's secondary grade, which is also ranked from 1 to 5. These two grades are added together to determine the total Gleason score. For example, a primary grade of 3 and a secondary grade of 4, when combined, equal a Gleason score of 7 (a moderately aggressive cancer).

Another, less common, technique for determining the aggressiveness of prostate cancer is called the Mostofi grading system, which uses Roman numerals to rank the cancer's aggressiveness. Grade I is equal to a Gleason score of 2-4, grade II is equal to a Gleason score of 5-7, and grade III is equal to a Gleason score of 8-10.

Table 5A — What a Gleason Score Actually Means

Your total Gleason score makes a big difference in telling how your cancer may progress. Cancers with a Gleason score of 2-4 do not usually spread beyond the prostate within 10 years, while half of those in the 5-7 range may do so. Cancers with a score in the 8-10 range are the most aggressive; most escape the prostate within a decade.

Gleason Score	Mostofi Score	What does the pathologist call it?	What does that actually mean?	In 10 years, what is the chance that this cancer will leave my prostate and enter other parts of my body?
2-4	I	"A well-differentiated prostate cancer"	Cancer cells are uniform in shape and close together	25%
5-7	II	"A moderately differentiated prostate cancer"	Cancer cells have more irregular shapes and sizes	50%
8-10	III	"A poorly differentiated prostate cancer"	Cancer cells are lumped together in larger masses and are invading nearby connective tissue.	75%

FAST FACT

The majority (95 percent) of prostate cancers are called adenocarcinomas ("adeno" means gland; "carcinoma" means cancer). Less than 5 percent of all prostate cancers are non-adenocarcinomas, which are usually much more aggressive and do not respond to any type of hormonal treatment. (For more about hormonal therapy, see Chapter 8.)

So far, only one of the two vital questions about your prostate cancer has been answered: how aggressive, or fast-growing, it is. The next question that needs to be addressed is how far it has spread — what is the stage of the cancer? The answer will significantly affect the way your cancer can be treated.

B

What are the ABCD and TNM staging systems?

All prostate cancers have one thing in common: They start as a small tumor within the prostate gland. Some prostate tumors grow very slowly and stay within the prostate for many years, while others spread beyond the gland in just a short time.

After the diagnosis of prostate cancer, a host of questions must be answered: Is the cancer still confined to the prostate? Has it migrated to other reproductive organs next to the prostate? Has it spread to the lymph nodes? Has it traveled to the bones or other parts of the body?

To determine how far the cancer has spread, or "metastasized," you must undergo a series of tests. This is called the "staging" process. Once all the results are in, your cancer is assigned a "stage" using one of two methods (see Table 5B and Fig. 5B).

The Whitmore-Jewett, or ABCD, staging system — This method assigns the cancer a letter from A to D. A or B means the cancer is confined to the prostate, C or D indicates it has spread beyond the prostate or throughout the body. Stages A or B, quite obviously, are easier to treat than C or D. While this staging system is the oldest, it is still used by many doctors.

The TNM staging system — Thanks to the development of more sophisticated diagnostic tests, the TNM staging system was created. It provides an even more detailed picture than the Whitmore-Jewett method of how far the cancer has spread. The T stands for "tumor," the N is for "nodes" (as in lymph nodes) and the M is for "metastasis," or distant spreading of the cancer.

TNM staging results can be interpreted as follows:

T — When your tumor is staged, your report will include a capital T (for tumor) with a number (between 1 and 4) and a lower-case letter (a, b or c) next to it. The greater the number and letter, the farther the cancer has spread. For example, a T2c cancer is confined to the prostate but covers more areas of the gland than a T2a cancer. A T3c cancer has spread a little beyond the prostate, while a T4a cancer has spread far beyond the gland.

N — If the lymph nodes contain cancer, the staging report will also include a capital N (for nodes) with a plus sign next to it: "N + ."

M — If the cancer has spread far beyond the prostate — to the bones, for example — then the staging report will include a capital M (for metastasis) with a plus sign next to it: "M + ."

So, a staging report always includes a capital T with a number and lower-case letter following it, regardless whether the cancer is confined to the prostate or if it is advanced. The report may or may not include a capital N or M, because these letters only appear in reports that indicate the cancer has spread beyond the prostate to the lymph Nodes or other areas of the body (Metastasis).

Some doctors use both the ABCD and TNM staging systems, while other doctors use one or the other. Therefore, it is still important to understand both systems.

Getting doctors to convert from the traditional ABCD staging system to the newer TNM method is similar to getting most Americans to use the metric system. Although the metric system is more accurate, we are slow to accept it because we've been using the old measurement system for so long.

FAST FACT

Most people assume that prostate cancer begins growing in a single spot within the gland. In reality, the average cancerous prostate starts with seven different malignant spots and progresses from there. So, prostate cancer is really "multifocal," which means it starts growing in a variety of separate areas within the gland.

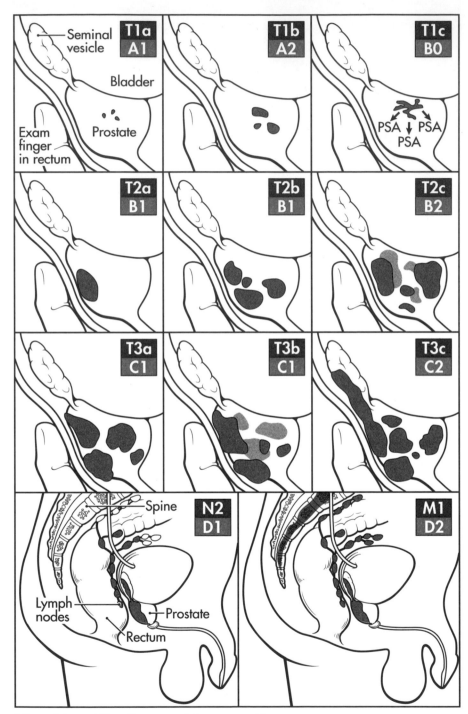

Fig. 5B — The Stages of Prostate Cancer

The progression of prostate cancer, from the earliest stages to the most advanced, along with the corresponding TNM and ABCD stages.

*Table 5B — The TNM and ABCD Staging Systems
and What They Mean*

TNM	ABCD	What the Results Mean
TO	—	No cancer.
T1a	A1	A cancer that is found during another procedure, such as TURP. The cancer takes up less than 5% of prostate tissue removed in the procedure.
T1b	A2	A cancer that is not felt by DRE or detected by PSA, but is found during a procedure such as TURP. The cancer takes up more than 5% of the prostate tissue removed in the procedure.
T1c	B0	A cancer that cannot be felt with DRE but is detected because of a high PSA level.
T2a	B1	A cancer that occupies 50% or less of one prostate lobe.
T2b	B1	A cancer that occupies more than 50% of one prostate lobe.
T2c	B2	A cancer that occupies any percentage of both prostate lobes.
T3a	C1	A cancer on one side of the prostate that is now growing on the outside and going beyond the prostate.
T3b	C1	A cancer on both sides of the prostate that is now growing on the outside and going beyond the prostate.
T3c	C2	A cancer that has invaded one or both seminal vesicles.
T4a	C2	A cancer that has spread to/invaded the bladder neck and/or external sphincter and/or rectum.
T4b	C2	A cancer that has invaded other areas near the prostate.
N0	—	No lymph nodes near the prostate have been invaded by cancer.
N1 (N+)	D1	A cancer that has metastasized/spread to one or more lymph nodes (2 cm or smaller).
N2 (N+)	D1	A cancer that has metastasized/spread to one or more lymph nodes (between 2 cm and 5 cm).
N3 (N+)	D1	A cancer that has spread to at least one lymph node (5 cm or larger).
M0	—	The cancer has not spread far beyond the prostate or local lymph nodes.
M1 (M+)	D2	The cancer has spread far beyond the prostate or local lymph nodes (to the bones, liver or lungs, for example).

C

What tests might I need to see whether my cancer has spread?

Determining the exact stage of your cancer is critical; your treatment decision depends on it. There are many tests that can be used to find out how far prostate cancer has spread. However, the only widely used test is the bone scan. Other tests, such as the chest X-ray, CT and MRI scan, rarely provide additional information, so their use is not recommended routinely. Below is a list of all the staging tests, from the least to the most invasive (see Fig. 5C):

Chest X-ray — This test is used to help determine whether the cancer has spread to the lungs. While less than 5 percent of all prostate cancers find their way to the lungs, about 25 percent of the advanced cases migrate there. Two X-ray pictures usually are taken, one from the front and one from the side. This is a harmless procedure, because the amount of radiation received is small.

CAT (computed axial tomography) scan — A CAT scan, commonly called a CT scan, is much more sensitive than an ordinary X-ray. It produces detailed, cross-sectional images of the body. When these images are electronically stacked on top of each other and shown on a computer screen, the doctor may view a specific part of the body and its surrounding structures from every angle.

When getting a CT scan, you will be asked to lie down on a narrow table that moves backward and forward. This table will slide you through the middle of a big, donut-shaped machine. As you lie there, the machine will take a series of pictures of your prostate and the area around it. The CT scan only lasts for a few minutes. Also, you may have an iodine-based solution (a contrast material) injected into an arm vein during the procedure to help the pictures come out better. As the IV solution goes in, you temporarily may feel a rush of heat throughout your body, but it is not painful. People who are allergic to iodine can still have a CT scan without the use of a contrast solution.

MRI (magnetic resonance imaging) scan — MRI uses magnetism and radio waves rather than X-rays or contrast dyes to produce a series of pictures. An MRI is usually much more expensive than a CT scan.

The MRI procedure requires you to lie within a small, tube-shaped device for 30 to 45 minutes. If you are uncomfortable being enclosed in such a small space, try to take a nap during this procedure. If you don't think you can sleep, ask your doctor if you can listen to music.

In various studies, CT and MRI have been shown to correctly stage only three to four out of 10 men (30 percent to 40 percent) with early, organ-confined disease. The test's accuracy increases only slightly for those with advanced prostate cancer. So, when it comes to prostate cancer, an MRI or a CT scan is of value only in determining whether the cancer has spread to the lymph nodes. Organ-confined prostate cancers can be very difficult to see on an MRI or CT scan because they are often tiny, peppered sparsely throughout the gland. Only when the cancer has formed a large mass or lump can it be detected through these high-tech imaging systems. Prostate cancer can be found much more accurately with a digital-rectal exam and a PSA blood test — for a fraction of the cost.

Bone scan (radionuclide scintigraphy) — A bone scan can find advanced prostate cancer (metastasis) better than any other test. However, research has shown that if a person recently diagnosed with prostate cancer has no skeletal pain and a PSA value of 10 ng/ml or less, then a bone scan may not be necessary. That's because in such men, the risk of having cancer that has spread to the bones is almost zero. On the other hand, if you are diagnosed with prostate cancer, it can be useful to have a bone scan right away so that any later bone scans can be compared to the first one, thus allowing your doctor to get a very good idea of your cancer's progress.

Before having a bone scan, which is similar to getting an X-ray, a harmless solution is injected into the bloodstream. This solution travels throughout the body and is attracted to areas where any bone changes may have occurred. The greater the change in the bones, the more solution is absorbed by that particular area. The solution is absorbed not only by cancerous areas but also by parts of the bone that have been affected by arthritis, fracture, infection or other types of disease, such as Pagets' disease. Therefore, a bone scan can be difficult to interpret in some individuals. However, this high degree of sensitivity is also its best feature.

When reading a bone scan, one side of the body should be compared to the other. If a dark spot (also called a hot spot) appears on both sides of the body in the same area, it is usually not cancer. However, if a spot appears on one side of the body, such as the right hip bone, but is not mirrored on the opposite side, this could be a sign of cancer. Other areas that do not have an equivalent location on the opposite side of the body, such as the bladder, can appear dark, or "hot," normally (see Fig. 5C).

Before reading about the next two procedures, please note that many doctors today do not use them if they already are given adequate information about the stage of the patient's prostate cancer from the Gleason score, PSA and digital-rectal examination.

Laparoscopic pelvic lymphadenectomy — Usually men who are at risk of having their localized prostate cancer spread quickly beyond the prostate (those with a high PSA level or Gleason score) are good candidates for this procedure, for it is the best way to see if there is any cancer in the lymph nodes.

You are usually put to sleep (general anesthesia) during this procedure, in which the doctor makes several tiny punctures on the abdomen. Using long surgical instruments and a special fiber-optic video camera, the doctor removes the pelvic lymph nodes through these small puncture sites. The lymph nodes are then analyzed to see if they contain cancer. There is only a short hospital stay associated with this procedure (one to two days) and you can usually return to work within a week.

Although this procedure is less invasive than standard open surgery, it could still be dangerous if you have a history of health problems, so make sure your doctor knows of any past abdominal surgeries or medical problems before undergoing this operation.

Staging pelvic lymphadenectomy, or minilaparotomy ("mini-lap") — The "minilap" procedure is similar to the laparoscopic pelvic lymphadenectomy except that a single larger, 3-inch incision is made. If there is cancer in the lymph nodes, this incision is closed and the procedure is concluded. If there is no cancer in the lymph nodes, some doctors will then extend the incision to the pubic bone and proceed with a radical retropubic prostatectomy (complete removal of the prostate) while you are still asleep, if that is your predetermined treatment choice.

Once you know the PSA value, Gleason score and TNM or ABCD stage of your prostate cancer, you will be able to make a good prediction, based on solid international research, of where your cancer is located and how it may progress (see Table 5C-1). This information will, in turn help you make a more well-informed treatment decision (see Table 5C-2).

CT Scan

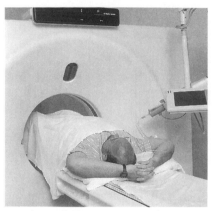

Patient being scanned

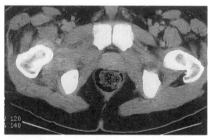

Normal CT

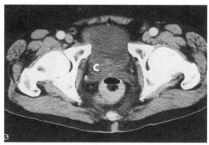

Abnormal CT

MRI Scan

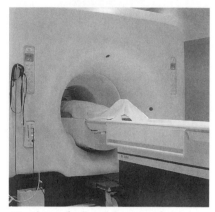

Patient being scanned

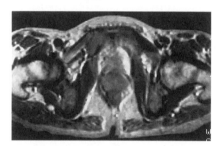

Normal MRI

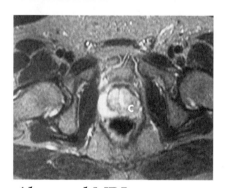

Abnormal MRI

Fig. 5C — Staging Tests for Prostate Cancer

The different tests used to determine the stage of your cancer, with examples of what a positive and a negative result would look like from each test. The best of these four tests is the bone scan. Depending on where you go to have your cancer staged, the other three tests may or may not be used.
(C=cancer, P=prostate, H=hip, B=bladder, L=left side of the body).

Bone Scan

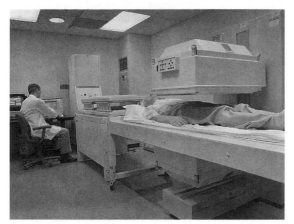

Patient being scanned

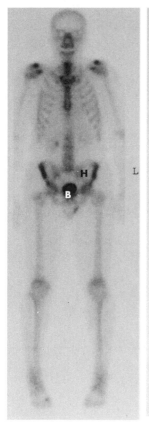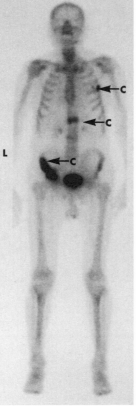

Normal
bone scan   *Abnormal*
bone scan

Chest X-ray

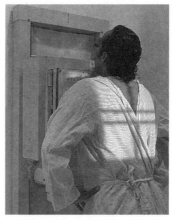

Patient being scanned

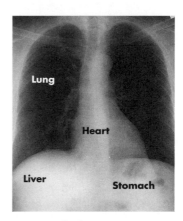

Normal chest X-ray

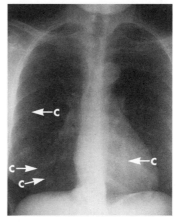

Abnormal chest X-ray

Table 5C-1— Determining How Far Your Cancer Has Spread (Based on PSA Value, Total Gleason Score and Clinical Stage)

	\multicolumn{7}{c}{PSA (ng/ml) 0.0-4.0}						
Score	\multicolumn{7}{c}{**Clinical Stage**}						
	T1a	T1b	T1c	T2a	T2b	T2c	T3a
	\multicolumn{7}{c}{*Prediction of organ-confined disease*}						
2-4	100	85	92	88	76	82	-
5	100	78	81	81	67	73	-
6	100	68	69	72	54	60	42
7	-	54	55	61	41	46	-
8-10	-	-	-	48	31	-	-
	T1a	T1b	T1c	T2a	T2b	T2c	T3a
	\multicolumn{7}{c}{*Prediction of established capsular penetration*}						
2-4	0	15	22	14	26	17	-
5	0	22	30	20	34	26	-
6	0	30	34	29	46	38	59
7	-	43	40	39	59	50	-
8-10	-	-	-	50	68	-	-
	T1a	T1b	T1c	T2a	T2b	T2c	T3a
	\multicolumn{7}{c}{*Prediction of seminal vesicle involvement*}						
2-4	0	1	< 1	1	2	2	-
5	0	3	< 1	2	4	4	-
6	0	6	1	5	9	9	8
7	-	12	4	9	17	17	-
8-10	-	-	-	17	29	-	-
	T1a	T1b	T1c	T2a	T2b	T2c	T3a
	\multicolumn{7}{c}{*Prediction of lymph nodal involvement*}						
2-4	0	2	< 1	1	2	4	-
5	0	4	1	2	4	8	-
6	0	8	2	3	9	17	15
7	-	15	2	7	18	31	-
8-10	-	-	-	13	32	-	-

Numbers represent probability (%). Dash represents lack of sufficient data to calculate probability.

Table 5C-1 (cont'd)

Score	T1a	T1b	T1c	T2a	T2b	T2c	T3a
PSA (ng/ml) 4.1-10							
Clinical Stage							
Prediction of organ-confined disease							
2-4	100	78	82	83	67	71	-
5	100	70	71	73	56	64	43
6	100	53	59	62	44	48	33
7	100	39	43	51	32	37	26
8-10	-	32	31	39	22	25	12
	T1a	T1b	T1c	T2a	T2b	T2c	T3a
Prediction of established capsular penetration							
2-4	0	22	29	19	34	27	-
5	0	29	34	28	45	34	58
6	0	45	38	38	56	49	68
7	0	58	44	49	68	59	75
8-10	-	64	48	59	77	71	87
	T1a	T1b	T1c	T2a	T2b	T2c	T3a
Prediction of seminal vesicle involvement							
2-4	0	2	< 1	1	3	3	-
5	0	4	< 1	3	6	6	5
6	0	9	1	6	11	12	11
7	0	18	5	12	22	23	18
8-10	-	29	23	22	38	40	40
	T1a	T1b	T1c	T2a	T2b	T2c	T3a
Prediction of lymph nodal involvement							
2-4	0	2	1	1	2	5	-
5	0	4	1	2	5	10	8
6	0	9	2	4	11	19	16
7	0	18	3	8	20	34	28
8-10	-	30	5	15	35	53	50

Numbers represent probability (%). Dash represents lack of sufficient data to calculate probability.

Table 5C-1 (cont'd)

Score	PSA (ng/ml) 10.1-20						
	Clinical Stage						
	T1a	T1b	T1c	T2a	T2b	T2c	T3a
	Prediction of organ-confined disease						
2-4	100	-	-	61	52	-	-
5	100	49	55	58	43	37	26
6	-	36	41	44	28	37	19
7	-	24	24	36	19	24	14
8-10	-	11	-	29	14	15	9
	T1a	T1b	T1c	T2a	T2b	T2c	T3a
	Prediction of established capsular penetration						
2-4	0	-	-	40	49	-	-
5	0	49	40	43	58	61	75
6	-	62	45	56	73	59	82
7	-	73	52	64	81	73	86
8-10	-	87	-	70	86	82	92
	T1a	T1b	T1c	T2a	T2b	T2c	T3a
	Prediction of seminal vesicle involvement						
2-4	0	-	-	3	4	-	-
5	0	7	< 1	5	8	12	11
6	-	15	1	11	19	17	18
7	-	28	6	19	33	33	31
8-10	-	55	-	29	50	53	49
	T1a	T1b	T1c	T2a	T2b	T2c	T3a
	Prediction of lymph nodal involvement						
2-4	0	-	-	1	3	-	-
5	0	5	3	2	6	13	11
6	-	11	4	5	13	22	20
7	-	21	7	9	24	39	35
8-10	-	41	-	17	40	59	54

Numbers represent probability (%). Dash represents lack of sufficient data to calculate probability.

Table 5C-1 (cont'd)

Score				Clinical Stage			
	T1a	T1b	T1c	T2a	T2b	T2c	T3a

PSA (ng/ml) Greater than 20

Prediction of organ-confined disease

Score	T1a	T1b	T1c	T2a	T2b	T2c	T3a
2-4	-	-	33	20	7	-	-
5	-	-	24	32	-	3	-
6	-	-	22	14	11	4	5
7	-	-	7	18	4	5	3
8-10	-	-	3	3	1	2	2

Prediction of established capsular penetration

Score	T1a	T1b	T1c	T2a	T2b	T2c	T3a
2-4	-	-	50	80	94	-	-
5	-	-	54	68	-	97	-
6	-	-	53	86	90	96	95
7	-	-	67	80	96	95	98
8-10	-	-	74	97	99	97	98

Prediction of seminal vesicle involvement

Score	T1a	T1b	T1c	T2a	T2b	T2c	T3a
2-4	-	-	< 1	12	30	-	-
5	-	-	< 1	11	-	29	-
6	-	-	2	35	40	53	31
7	-	-	9	31	73	62	55
8-10	-	-	81	81	93	73	65

Prediction of lymph nodal involvement

Score	T1a	T1b	T1c	T2a	T2b	T2c	T3a
2-4	-	-	6	2	7	-	-
5	-	-	9	3	-	29	-
6	-	-	8	9	18	53	31
7	-	-	24	11	44	62	55
8-10	-	-	41	35	76	73	65

Numbers represent probability (%). Dash represents lack of sufficient data to calculate probability.

Table 5C-2 — Possible Treatment Options for Prostate Cancer (with Respect to Stage)

Clinical Disease Name	Stage	Options
Localized	A, B, T1, T2	Cryotherapy External-beam radiation therapy Radical prostatectomy Radioactive-seed implants Watchful waiting
Locally advanced (Just beyond the prostate)	C, T3, T4	Cryotherapy External-beam radiation therapy Hormone therapy Radioactive-seed implants
Advanced, or metastasized, to the lymph nodes and bone	D, N+, M+	Chemotherapy Hormone therapy Spot radiation/strontium/ medications for pain

FAST FACT

The clinical stage of prostate cancer is an estimation of how far the disease has spread based on a variety of tests, from a digital-rectal exam to a bone scan. The pathological stage is based on a pathologist's evaluation of the radical prostatectomy specimen. The pathological stage is more accurate, but it can only be determined after the prostate has been surgically removed.

The ABCs of CHAPTER 5

A Quick Review

A

What is the Gleason grading system?

- Because not all prostate cancers look or act the same, it must be "graded" by a pathologist, which tells your doctor how aggressive your cancer is. This helps you and your doctor decide on the proper course of treatment.

- The cancer is given an overall Gleason score of 2-10; the lower the score, the more responsive the cancer is to treatment. A score in the middle range (5-7), also called the "gray zone," means that the cancer usually varies in its ability to be treated successfully.

- Some low-score prostate cancers (2-4) are associated with a significant increase in PSA level, while some high-score prostate cancers (8-10) are not linked with a markedly high PSA blood level.

B

What are the ABCD and TNM staging systems?

- Staging your prostate cancer allows you and your doctor to know how far your cancer has spread, which has a significant impact on your treatment options.

- Two staging systems are used today: the Whitmore-Jewett, or ABCD system, which is the oldest and most widely used method in this country; and the TNM staging system, which is newer, more informative and gaining acceptance.

- If your cancer is stage A or B, or if it is a T1 or T2, then it has not spread beyond the prostate. If your cancer is a stage C or D, or if it is a T3 or T4 (or N+ and/or M+), then your cancer has spread beyond the prostate.

C

What tests might I need to see whether my cancer has spread?

- A chest X-ray, a CT scan and an MRI are of little value when it comes to staging prostate cancer.

- A bone scan is very sensitive and is a very good indicator of cancer spread to the skeleton, especially when the PSA level is greater than 10 ng/ml.

- Either a laparoscopic pelvic lymphadenectomy or a "minilap" may be useful to see whether the cancer has spread to the lymph nodes, but many physicians who are able to clinically stage a man's prostate cancer from the Gleason score, PSA and rectal exam choose not to use either procedure for further staging information.

Medical References

Title: **"Eliminating the need for bilateral pelvic lymphadenectomy in select patients with prostate cancer"**
Authors: Bluestein, D.L.; Bostwick, D.G.; Bergstralh, E.J.; et al
Journal: *Journal of Urology*
Volume: 151
Pages: 1315-1320
Date: May 1994

Title: **"PSA-detected (clinical stage T1c or Bo) prostate cancer. Pathologically significant tumors."**
Authors: Oesterling, J.E.; Suman, V.J.; Zincke, H.; et al
Journal: *Urology Clinics of North America*
Volume: 20 (4)
Pages: 687-693
Date: November 1993

Title: **"The use of prostate-specific antigen in staging patients with newly diagnosed prostate cancer"**
Authors: Oesterling, J.E.; Martin, S.K.; Bergstralh, E.J.; et al
Journal: *Journal of the American Medical Association (JAMA)*
Volume: 269
Pages: 57-60
Date: Jan. 6, 1993

Title: **"Comparison of magnetic resonance imaging and ultrasonography in staging early prostate cancer. Results of a multi-institutional cooperative trial."**
Authors: Rifkin, M.D.; Zerhouni, E.A.; Gatsonis, C.A.; et al
Journal: *New England Journal of Medicine*
Volume: 323 (10)
Pages: 621-626
Date: Sept. 6, 1990

Title: **"The definition and preoperative prediction of clinically insignificant prostate cancer"**
Authors: Dugan, J.A.; Bostwick, D.G.; Myers, R.P.; et al
Journal: *Journal of the American Medical Association (JAMA)*
Volume: 275 (4)
Pages: 288-294
Date: Jan. 24-31, 1996

Notes

6

The Cancer is Confined to the Prostate: Traditional Treatments

A

Can nontreatment really
be an option?

B

Is radiation therapy
for me?

C

What are the pros and
cons of surgery?

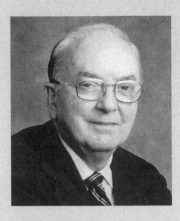

Jesse Helms
U.S. senator

The dangerous reality of prostate cancer has struck a number of us here on Capitol Hill. Fortunately for me, surgery was not necessary — I underwent radiation therapy every morning for 39 days. It goes without saying that I am thankful for early detection and am convinced that it was the key to my recovered health.

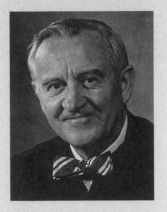

Paul Stevens
U.S. Supreme Court justice

During a routine physical examination my doctor told me that my PSA was abnormally high and recommended that I consult a urologist. A biopsy determined that I was positive for cancer. Fortunately, the cancer had been detected early and was confined, or localized.

At the age of 71, I gave serious consideration to two treatment options: radical prostatectomy and radiation (the third option, watchful waiting, I did not consider seriously). After discussing these options with three different doctors and with friends who had been treated for prostate cancer, I decided on radiation treatment.

In six or seven weeks my treatment was completed and, I believe, was entirely successful. I was also very happy with this treatment choice because it did not significantly affect my lifestyle. I am still able to go to work every day and exercise regularly.

I did experience some dizziness at the end of the treatment, but that lasted for only an hour or so.

Given the prevalence of prostate cancer, I strongly believe in frequent checkups to detect the disease while it is still amenable to treatment.

A

Can nontreatment really be an option?

For some men diagnosed with prostate cancer, there is an alternative to medical and surgical treatment. It is called "watchful waiting." Sometimes it is also called "surveillance," "observation," "expectant therapy," "expectant management" or "deferred treatment."

Again, as was mentioned in Chapter 4, watchful waiting does not mean that you and your doctor sit back and do nothing. It means that even though you've decided not to have treatment, your prostate cancer is still being regularly monitored through PSA testing, digital-rectal exams and/or transrectal ultrasounds (see Fig. 6A). (The word "regular" here means that you should return at least every six months to see how your cancer is doing. The doctor also may want to do a biopsy once a year or more to get a better idea of the cancer's aggressiveness.) And it means that as soon as any changes are detected through any of these diagnostic tests, you can still go ahead with active treatment.

The best candidates for watchful waiting are:
- men whose life expectancy is no more than 10 years due to age (such as those over 75), illness or genetic history;
- men over the age of 70 with a well-differentiated (Gleason score of 2-4), very small cancer;
- men whose cancer is confined to the prostate and who want to take time to decide what type of treatment they may have; and
- men who have advanced prostate cancer (cancer that has spread beyond the prostate gland) and have not experienced symptoms.

The advantages of watchful waiting:
- You can avoid side effects or complications associated with any of the treatments for prostate cancer.
- It is the least expensive option in the short term. The only costs associated with this management approach involve regular PSA testing, digital-rectal exams and occasional prostate biopsies,

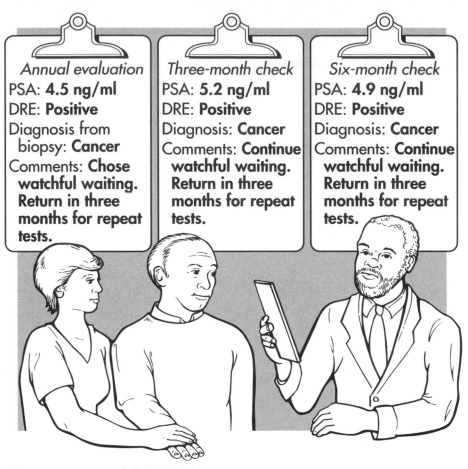

Fig. 6A — Watchful Waiting

Watchful waiting is an active process that involves regular prostate check-ups to monitor the cancer.

which total about $1,200 a year. However, if your prostate cancer should spread, then the long-term costs of treatment could easily outweigh the short-term savings.

• It can give you time to make a calm and rational treatment decision with your family and your doctor. Prostate cancer can be a very slow-growing malignancy. When it is confined to the prostate it can take several years for it to double in size. Therefore, even though it is a gamble, you may have time to reap the benefits of watchful waiting.

The disadvantage of watchful waiting:

IT ALLOWS THE CANCER TO CONTINUE TO GROW. And even for cancers that are not aggressive or large, it can still be a risk because any cancer can change its characteristics at any time. A cancer that has a Gleason score of 4 today could develop into a 5 or 7 practically overnight.

A report in the *New England Journal of Medicine* that summarized a number of studies on watchful waiting found that among those who opted against treatment, almost half experienced cancer growth beyond the prostate within 10 years. It is a fact that physicians cannot predict how fast a cancer will grow or if it will become more aggressive with time. It is also possible that a cancer can go from a curable state to an incurable state without a noticeable change in PSA level, digital-rectal exam or transrectal ultrasound results.

Among men with a Gleason score of 2-4, about 2 percent develop cancer outside the prostate gland within the first year of watchful waiting. In the second year, 4 percent of these men develop metastases (advanced cancer). The number increases by 2 percent each additional year. Among men with a Gleason score of 7-10, about 14 percent develop metastatic cancer during the first year of watchful waiting. The number increases by 14 percent each year thereafter. The yearly risk of cancer metastasis among men with a Gleason score in the middle range (5-6) is not known.

For a summary of all the research studies on watchful waiting completed from 1966 to 1993, see Table 6A. The patients represented in this table had organ-confined prostate cancer.

A note on conservatively treated localized prostate cancer: A recent study from the *Journal of the American Medical Association* looked at men aged 65-75 years old receiving immediate or delayed hormonal (drug) therapy only for localized prostate cancer and found the following results:

• Men with a Gleason score of 2-4 lived as long as men in the normal population without prostate cancer.

- Men with a Gleason score of 5-7 lived four to five years less than men without prostate cancer.
- Men with a Gleason score of 8-10 lived six to eight years less than men without prostate cancer.

These results indicate that watchful waiting is an adequate treatment option for older men with low-grade cancers (Gleason score 2-4). However, older men with moderate (Gleason score 5-7) or high grade cancer (Gleason score 8-10) should consider receiving some kind of treatment.

*Table 6A — The Effectiveness of Watchful Waiting on Localized Prostate Cancer**

	After 5 years	After 10 years	After 15 years
Percentage of men still alive *(overall survival)*:	67-92%	34-71%	39-67%
Percentage of men who have not died of prostate cancer *(disease-specific or cause-specific survival)*:	89-99%	84-85%	68%
Percentage of men whose cancer has progressed *(metastasis)*:	32%	47%	unknown

*Organ-confined (T2) cancer only

Average patient age: 70 years

Total number of patients evaluated: 913

Cancer characteristics of these patients: 62% had well-differentiated, 35% had moderately differentiated and 3% had poorly differentiated malignancies.

Source: *Journal of Urology*, Volume 154, Pages 2144-2148, December 1995.

FAST FACT

One in 10 men (10 percent) diagnosed with prostate cancer will choose watchful waiting instead of medical or surgical treatment.

B

Is radiation therapy for me?

The primary type of radiation therapy used to treat prostate cancer is called "external-beam radiation therapy." This is just a fancy way of saying that you will be receiving radiation from what looks like a big X-ray machine. The machine very accurately delivers radiation through the pelvis to the prostate. Radiation therapy is quick and painless, but it does involve going to the hospital five days a week for approximately seven weeks. Each treatment session lasts about 15 to 30 minutes.

Many institutions use a CT scan of your pelvis to accurately show technicians and doctors the exact location of your organs. A computer is then used to calculate the best possible positions the external beam can be targeted to most accurately deliver the radiation to the prostate (see Fig. 6B-1). During treatment, you are asked to lie down on a table while the machine changes positions around the table. A variety of beam angles ensures the most effective treatment (see Fig. 6B-2).

Today, you do not have to worry about receiving radiation in an area that does not need it, because lead blocks protect those sites. Regardless of whether your cancer has spread beyond the prostate, you will receive radiation not only to the prostate but to the areas around it.

Radiation therapy can be used for men of any age with any stage of cancer. Therefore, the best candidates for this treatment are:

- men who are expected to live at least 10 more years;
- men whose cancer is confined to the prostate;
- men who cannot be cured by surgery — those whose cancer has already escaped the prostate at the time of diagnosis or men whose cancer has returned after initial surgical treatment; and
- men who do not want to be treated with surgery.

Advantages of radiation therapy:

- The outcome for patients with localized cancer is similar to that of radical prostatectomy (surgical removal of the prostate). Between 40 percent and 60 percent of patients with both localized and advanced cancer are alive 15 years after treatment.

- It is done on an outpatient basis; after your clinic visit, you can go home.

Disadvantages of radiation therapy (see Table 6B-2):

- It is difficult afterward for doctors to tell if you have really been cured, because a low PSA level after radiation therapy does not always guarantee total elimination of the prostate cancer.

- The cancer cannot be pathologically staged (the prostate is not removed, so it cannot be examined by a pathologist).

- There are complications associated with radiation therapy. These side effects usually develop toward the end of the treatment, or even months after the therapy has ended.

- It is expensive, with an average total cost of between $10,000 and $30,000.

Complications associated with radiation therapy (from most to least common):

Sexual or erectile dysfunction — The majority of men who receive radiation therapy do not have problems with erections or intercourse in the short term. However, depending on which study you read, almost 30 percent of men receiving radiation can have some sexual complications in the long run.

Because some of the best candidates for radiation therapy are older men, and because some degree of sexual dysfunction goes hand in hand with increased age, it is hard to say exactly how strongly radiation affects sexual function. Studies show that less than 10 years after undergoing radiation therapy, 30 percent of men will have sexual or erectile difficulty. But statistics also tell us that the younger you are the better your chance of retaining sexual function after radiation, and if your cancer has not spread beyond the prostate, the better your chance of maintaining normal sexual activity. However, a younger man whose cancer is confined to the

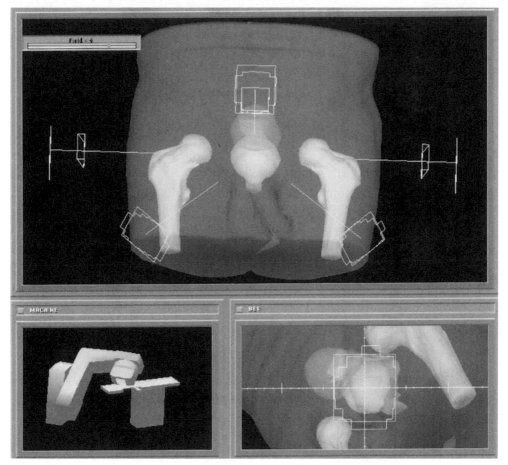

Fig. 6B-1 — External-beam Radiation Therapy Planning

These photos show the computer model that determines the most effective radiation-beam angles for treatment.

prostate will likely opt for surgery (or radioactive-seed implants) instead of radiation therapy because it offers as good or greater a chance of long-term cure.

Bowel complications — Diarrhea, rectal pain and the feeling of constantly wanting to have a bowel movement are the most common bowel complications associated with radiation therapy. However, in large studies involving more than 1,000 men receiving radiation therapy, the incidence of chronic bowel complications was approximately 5 percent.

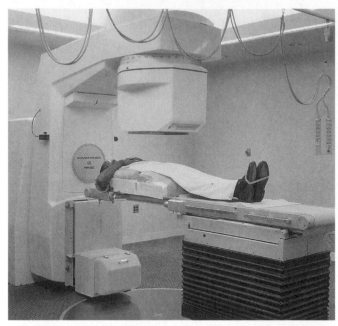

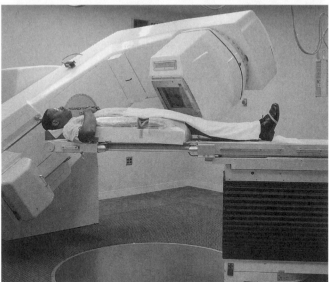

Fig. 6B-2 — External-beam Radiation Therapy Delivery

The actual delivery of external-beam radiation therapy from different angles. The treatment takes between 15 and 30 minutes per session.

Urinary problems — You may leak urine, need to urinate often (especially at night), feel that you have to constantly urinate, or experience painful urination. Studies have shown that more than three out of four men (75 percent) who undergo radiation therapy will need some type of medication to help with urination while they are receiving treatment. However, less than 5 percent of men who undergo radiation experience urinary complications serious enough to require hospitalization. Less than 1 percent of those hospitalized require an operation to fix their problem.

The most common complaints among radiation patients are having to urinate more often and/or having blood in the urine. Complications requiring hospitalization include urethral strictures (narrowing or blockage of the urethra from scar tissue), bladder problems and/or bloody urine. The majority of such hospitalizations are among men who've had surgery for benign prostate enlargement prior to undergoing treatment for prostate cancer. Overall, approximately 5 percent will experience long-term complications.

For a summary of all the research studies completed on external-beam radiation therapy between 1966-1993, see Table 6B-1 on the next page. The patients represented in this table had organ-confined (T2) prostate cancer.

Table 6B-1 — The Effectiveness of External-beam Radiation Therapy for Localized Prostate Cancer*

	After 5 years	After 10 years	After 15 years
Percentage of men still alive *(overall survival)*:	51-93%	41-70%	31-33%
Percentage of men who have not died of prostate cancer *(disease-specific or cause-specific survival)*:	63-96%	66-86%	unknown
Percentage of men whose cancer has progressed *(metastasis)*:	7-68%	36-60%	unknown

*Organ-confined (T2) cancers only

Average patient age: 66 years

Total number of patients evaluated: 14,205

Cancer characteristics of these patients: 41% had well-differentiated, 41% had moderately differentiated and 18% had poorly differentiated tumors.

Source: *Journal of Urology*, Volume 154, Pages 2144-2148, December 1995.

Table 6B-2 — **Report Card:** *External-beam Radiation Therapy*

✔ **Effectiveness**	
15-year survival rate (localized and advanced)	40-60%
✔ **Side effects**	
Risk of impotence	20-30%
Risk of bladder injury	10-20%
Risk of rectal problems	10-20%
Risk of urinary incontinence	< 3%
Risk of treatment-related death	0.2%
✔ **Total average cost**	$10,000–$30,000

C

What are the pros and cons of surgery?

Until quite recently, up to 90 percent of men who underwent complete surgical removal of the prostate, or radical prostatectomy, were left with sagging sexual function and up to 20 percent became incontinent. The majority of patients also experienced significant blood loss during surgery, requiring several transfusions.

In the past decade, however, a more refined approach to prostate-removal surgery has become widespread. This "nerve-sparing" or "anatomical" approach, developed in the early 80s by Patrick Walsh, M.D., of Johns Hopkins, involves using long, thin surgical instruments to cut free and protect the nerves and valves surrounding the prostate that control sexual function and urination.

The ability to have an erection is controlled by nerve bundles located on each side of the prostate. Whether one or both of these nerve bundles can be spared during surgery depends on the extent and location of the cancer. If the cancer is located centrally, away from the outer surface of the gland, then both nerve bundles can be spared. If the cancer is on one side, then only one nerve bundle needs to be removed. If both sides of the prostate are cancerous, then both nerve bundles must go. The nerves on both sides also are traditionally removed in men who already suffer from impotence, or the inability to achieve an erection, at the time of surgery. Since their nerve bundles are no longer needed, it is not necessary to save them.

You can still have an erection if only one nerve bundle is removed. If both are removed, you can still have a normal sex drive, sensation and orgasm, but you cannot have a normal erection.

However, even if both sets of nerves have been removed, with the help of certain devices and medications you can achieve an erection as good as those you had naturally before surgery. (For more information about these interventions, see Chapter 9.)

It is important to note that after the prostate is removed, ejaculations will be "dry," which means very little fluid will come out. This is because the prostate and the seminal vesicles, which are removed during surgery, make most of the seminal fluid, which carries sperm from the testicles. Therefore, if you still want to have a child, then a needle aspiration of sperm from your testicles can be done. The sperm is then used for in-vitro fertilization. This technique has a 30-percent success rate at an average cost of $8,500 per attempt (not usually covered by insurance).

There are two types of nerve-sparing or anatomical radical prostatectomy (see Figs. 6C-1 and 6C-2):

Radical retropubic prostatectomy — This is the most common type of prostate-removal surgery, accounting for 85 percent of all such operations. In this procedure, a vertical incision is made about an inch above the penis (in front of the pubic bone) up to the navel, or belly button. At the beginning of the operation, the pelvic lymph nodes can be removed through this incision and examined to determine for certain whether the cancer has spread beyond the prostate. If the lymph nodes are clear, the operation continues. If they are cancerous, the operation is discontinued and other treatment methods are explored.

Radical perineal prostatectomy — An operation in which a semicircular incision is made between the scrotum (the pouch that holds the testicles) and the anus. If the pelvic lymph nodes need to be examined, a separate incision must be made in the lower abdomen. In general, there is less bleeding with this type of prostatectomy and heavier men fare better with this approach. Also, there is no visible scar in the abdominal area. However, it is more difficult to save the nerve bundles — and thus erectile function — with this type of surgery.

Regardless of which style of radical prostatectomy is chosen, the outcome and side effects depend largely on who is doing the surgery. That's why it is important to take your time when choosing a surgeon and pick one who has not only been properly trained but performs this surgery regularly. Whether you can be cured from

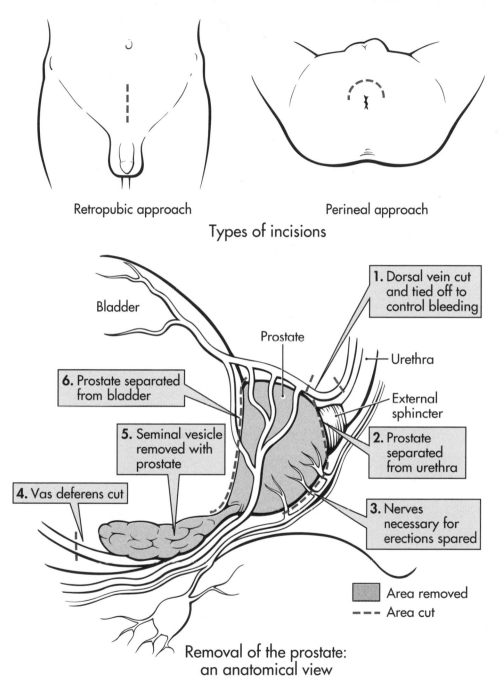

Retropubic approach   Perineal approach

Types of incisions

Bladder

Prostate

1. Dorsal vein cut and tied off to control bleeding

Urethra

6. Prostate separated from bladder

External sphincter

5. Seminal vesicle removed with prostate

2. Prostate separated from urethra

4. Vas deferens cut

3. Nerves necessary for erections spared

Area removed
--- Area cut

Removal of the prostate:
an anatomical view

*Fig. 6C-1 — The incisions used in the two types of radical prosta-
tectomy, the order in which the surgeon carries out the procedure,
and the final reconstruction process in the surgery, which takes
about three hours.*

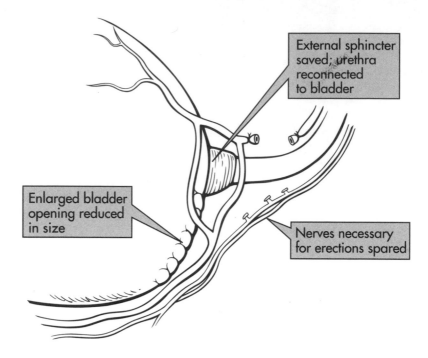

External sphincter saved; urethra reconnected to bladder

Enlarged bladder opening reduced in size

Nerves necessary for erections spared

Reconstruction of the
urinary tract

Fig. 6C-2 — Radical Prostatectomy (cont'd)

this operation depends also on the cancer's grade and stage. The earlier it is caught and the less aggressive it is, the better your chances of being cured.

If after surgery the PSA level increases or the cancer returns, then radiation therapy is still a treatment option.

The best candidates for radical prostatectomy are:

- men who are expected to live at least 10 more years (usually those under age 70); and
- men whose cancer is confined to prostate gland.

Those who DO NOT qualify for radical prostatectomy are:

- men with a life expectancy of less than 10 years;
- men who suffer from other serious medical conditions, such as congestive heart failure; and
- men whose cancer has spread beyond the prostate.

The advantages of radical prostatectomy:

- It can cure prostate cancer.
- It allows the cancer to be accurately staged through pathological examination of the tumor specimen.
- The PSA test can be used as an accurate predictor of whether the cancer has been completely removed or if it has returned.

Disadvantages of radical prostatectomy:

- It is a major operation; the recovery period is six to eight weeks.
- There is a small risk of significant blood loss, so you may wish to donate your own blood within the month before surgery in case a transfusion becomes necessary.

Prostatectomy also can result in a variety of postsurgical complications (see Table 6C-1), including:

Sexual or erectile dysfunction — This occurs in at least one in four individuals (25 percent), up to a maximum of three in four (75 percent). The degree of dysfunction is often related to age and the size of the cancer. Younger men and those with smaller tumors tend to have fewer sexual complications.

Incontinence (loss of urinary control) — Urinary incontinence occurs in 3 to greater than 50 percent of men. However, it may take six to nine months to regain urinary control.

Bowel complications — The number of men who experience rectal injury during surgery is less than 0.5 percent. If it should happen, the small defect can be fixed at the time of surgery with no long-term side effects.

For a summary of all the research studies that were completed on radical prostatectomy from 1966 to 1993, see Table 6C-2.

Table 6C-1 — **Report Card:** *Radical Prostatectomy*

✔ **Effectiveness**	
15-year survival rate (localized)	22-75 %
✔ **Side effects**	
Risk of impotence	50 %
Risk of surgical bleeding	< 5 %
Risk of urethral narrowing	< 5 %
Risk of rectal injury	< 1 %
Risk of urinary incontinence	3- > 50 %
Risk of treatment-related death	0.2 %
✔ **Total average cost**	$12,000–$15,000

Preparing for surgery: things you should know

- Stop using any products that could cause your blood to thin, such as aspirin, at least two weeks before the surgery to prevent excessive bleeding during the operation.

- You will need to have your rectum and part of your intestine cleared of any fecal material the night before surgery to reduce your chances of an infection. You will be given an enema or laxatives to assist with this process.

- You will be asked to decide between two types of anesthesia: general anesthesia, which puts you to sleep and is delivered in one dose; or epidural anesthesia, which numbs the area being operated on and can be delivered in more than one dose, according to your individual needs. Although there have been some reports that epidural anesthesia reduces the risk of developing blood clots in the legs, there has not been a formal study to prove or disprove this theory.

- Finally, it is important to know that if you have had. prior prostate surgery (as for BPH) then you must wait two to three months between procedures. This allows time for your prostate to heal before the additional surgery.

Table 6C-2 — The Effectiveness of Radical Prostatectomy for Localized Prostate Cancer*

	After 5 years	After 10 years	After 15 years
Percentage of men still alive *(overall survival)*:	69-95%	44-88%	22-75%
Percentage of men who have not died of prostate cancer *(disease-specific or cause-specific survival)*:	90-97%	88-93%	55-93%
Percentage of men whose cancer has progressed *(metastasis)*:	8-18%	18%	30%

*Organ-confined (T2) cancers only

Average patient age: 63 years

Total number of patients evaluated: 263

Cancer characteristics of these patients: 23% had well-differentiated, 57% had moderately differentiated, and 20% had poorly differentiated cancers.

Source: *Journal of Urology*, Volume 154, Pages 2144-2148, December 1995.

Recovering from surgery: what to expect

In the hospital:

- You will spend an average of three to seven days in the hospital.
- You will awake from surgery with a catheter in your penis, which drains urine from your bladder. This allows your urinary tract to rest and recover. The catheter must remain in place for two to three weeks, so you also will be wearing it home.
- You also will have one or two drainage tubes coming out of your lower abdomen, which prevents internal fluid buildup or infection. The tubes will be in place for about one to three days.
- You will be given pain medication (Ketorolac or Toradol), which, in addition to relieving your discomfort, should help stimulate your appetite within a few days.

- To prevent straining, you will be given a laxative to soften your stool and promote regular bowel movements. (Important: do not use an enema for at least six weeks after surgery.)

At home:

- Do not lift anything heavier than 10 pounds for six weeks after surgery.
- Do not drive a car for three weeks.
- Do not sit on a hard chair with a straight back for three weeks, or as long as the catheter is in place.
- Eat and drink whatever you want.
- Walk regularly to prevent blood clots from forming.
- In general, avoid any strenuous activity for at least six weeks after surgery to give your incision a chance to heal properly .

The ABCs of CHAPTER 6

A Quick Review

A

Can nontreatment really be an option?

- Watchful waiting doesn't mean sitting back and doing nothing. It means monitoring your cancer through regular PSA tests, digital-rectal exams and/or transrectal ultrasounds, as well as a possible annual biopsy.

- Those who qualify for watchful waiting are primarily men whose life expectancy is less than 10 years, either because of their age or other current health problems.

- The big advantages of watchful waiting are that you can avoid side effects related to the various treatments, and you can take some time before choosing a treatment option.

  The big disadvantage of watchful waiting is that it's a gamble; the window between having a curable cancer and an incurable one often closes silently.

Most cancers will spread beyond the prostate after 10 years; at this point the cancer is no longer curable.

B

Is radiation therapy for me?

- Men who qualify for radiation therapy are those with a life expectancy of less than 10 years, those who cannot be cured by surgery, those who've had a recurrence of cancer after surgery, or those who do not want surgery.

- The biggest advantage of external-beam radiation therapy is that it is not invasive like surgery.

- The biggest disadvantage of radiation therapy is that there can be bladder and rectal complications and problems with sexual function, such as difficulty having an erection.

C

What are the pros and cons of surgery?

- There are two types of surgery that allow the complete removal of the prostate while sparing the nerves that control erection: the retropubic radical prostatectomy (a vertical incision between the penis and navel) and the perineal radical prostatectomy (a semicircular incision between the scrotum and anus). The latter is well-suited for heavier men and causes less bleeding. However, it is more difficult for the surgeon to save the nerve bundles that preserve sexual function.

- Men who can benefit from surgery are those with a life expectancy greater than 10 years whose cancer is confined to the prostate.

- The two main disadvantages of surgery are (from most to least common): the loss of natural erectile function and the loss of urinary control. With recent advances in surgical technique, the risk of these complications has decreased significantly.

Medical References

Title: **"The treatment of prostate cancer by conventional radiation therapy: an analysis of long-term outcome"**
Authors: Zietman, A.L.; Coen, J.J.; Dallow, K.C.; et al
Journal: *International Journal of Radiation Oncology, Biology and Physiology*
Volume: 32 (2)
Pages: 287-292
Date: May 15, 1995

Title: **"Long-term (15 years) results after radical prostatectomy for clinically localized (stage T2c or lower) prostate cancer"**
Authors: Zincke, H.; Oesterling, J.E.; Blute, M.L.; et al
Journal: *Journal of Urology*
Volume: 152 (5 pt 2)
Pages: 1850-1857
Date: November 1994

Title: **"Results of conservative management of clinically localized prostate cancer"**
Authors: Chodak, G.W.; Thisted, R.A.; Gerber, G.S.; et al
Journal: *New England Journal of Medicine*
Volume: 330 (4)
Pages: 242-248
Date: Jan. 27, 1994

Title: **"Serum PSA after anatomic radical prostatectomy. The Johns Hopkins experience after 10 years"**
Authors: Partin, A.W.; Pound, C.R.; Clemens, J.Q.; et al
Journal: *Urology Clinics of North America*
Volume: 20 (4)
Pages: 713-725
Date: November 1993

Title: **"External beam radiation treatment for prostate cancer: still the gold standard"**
Author: Hanks, G.E.
Journal: *Oncology*
Volume: 6 (3)
Pages: 79-86, 89, 90-94 (discussion)
Date: March 1992

Notes _____

_____

_____

_____

_____

_____

_____

_____

_____

_____

_____

_____

_____

_____

_____

_____

_____

_____

_____

7

Experimental Treatments for Localized Prostate Cancer

A

How do I decide if an experimental approach may be right for me?

B

Does "freezing" the prostate really stop the cancer from spreading?

C

What are radioactive-seed implants?

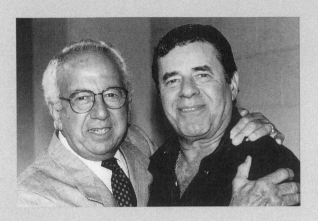

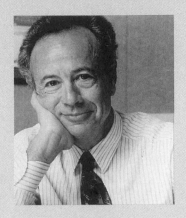

Jerry Lewis
Actor

I had a very small area in the prostate affected, found during my annual physical. Most doctors seem to agree that the safest procedure at the age of 65 is to totally remove the prostate to eliminate the possibility of spreading or recurrence, so I had the surgery. My doctors felt I could go without radiation.

I recovered completely, without any loss of function. I am now on a year's tour of "Damn Yankees," doing eight shows a week with time out to do the annual MDA Labor Day Telethon. I am proof that early detection is the key to successful treatment. I fully expect to live a long, healthy, productive life. I am now 70 years old!

Joe Stabile
Jerry Lewis' manager

I was 75 years old when my prostate cancer was discovered during my annual physical. The treatment we agreed upon was radiated seeds that were surgically implanted in the affected area of the prostate, followed by six weeks of daily radiation.

I am now 80 years old and in good health without any problems. I'm still playing tennis and water skiing and am still able to do my "homework!"

My advice is to get regular examinations — early detection is the key factor.

Andy Grove
Chief executive officer, Intel

As a result of my experience with prostate cancer, I've arrived at a few conclusions, including:

First, tumors grow. Sometimes they grow quickly, sometimes very slowly, but they do grow. I think you should hit a tumor with what you believe is your best shot, early and hard. In my case, it was a combination of hormones, high-dose-rate implant radiation and external radiation. For others, like Sen. Dole and Gen. Schwarzkopf, it was surgery. If my best friend had this disease, my advice to him would be, "Investigate, choose, and do — and do it quickly. Be aggressive now. Don't save the best for last."

Joe Stabile (left) and Jerry Lewis, above.

A
How do I decide if an experimental approach may be right for me?

The first thing you should do when considering any experimental procedure — or traditional treatment, for that matter — is to ask your doctor six general questions:

- Can you describe the treatment?
- Who are the best candidates for this approach?
- How effective is this treatment and what are its side effects?
- How much does the treatment cost, and would my insurance cover it?
- What are its advantages?
- What are its disadvantages?

But to get the best possible answers to the above questions, you must first ask the following specific questions (see Table 7A). Feel free to photocopy this list of questions and discuss the answers with your doctor or support group:

Table 7A — Questions to Ask Your Doctor About Experimental Treatment

---

1. If my cancer is confined to the prostate, how does this approach compare to the two most commonly used treatments — external-beam radiation therapy and radical prostatectomy (surgery)?

   ❑ Better   ❑ About the same   ❑ Not as good

2. If my cancer is not confined to the prostate, how does this treatment compare to external-beam radiation therapy, the most commonly used treatment for locally advanced cancer (cancer that has spread beyond the prostate to involve the neighboring tissues)?

   ❑ Better   ❑ About the same   ❑ Not as good

3. How long does the treatment take? _____

4. What is the average hospital stay?_____

5. What is the average cost of this treatment alone? _____

Table 7A — Questions to Ask Your Doctor (cont'd)

6. What is the total average cost, which includes all extra fees like hospitalization, X-rays and medication? _____

7. What percentage of the total cost will I have to pay? _____

8. What are the short-term (a year or less) and long-term side effects, in what percentage of patients do they occur and for how long, on average?

   ❑ **Erectile problems:**
        Percentage affected_____   How long_____

   ❑ **Urinary problems:**
        Percentage affected_____   How long_____

   ❑ **Bowel problems:**
        Percentage affected_____   How long_____

   ❑ **Other problems:**
        Percentage affected_____   How long_____

9. What precautions or lifestyle changes would be helpful to follow before and after treatment?

   Before treatment: _____

   _____

   _____

   After treatment: _____

   _____

   _____

10. What types of medications will I have to take before or after the treatment, and for how long?

    Before treatment
    Medication _____ Number of days _____
    Medication _____ Number of days _____
    Medication _____ Number of days _____

    After treatment
    Medication _____ Number of days _____
    Medication _____ Number of days _____
    Medication _____ Number of days _____

Table 7A — Questions to Ask Your Doctor (cont'd)

11.   Has this procedure been approved by the U.S. Food and Drug Administration, or FDA?
❑ Yes ❑ No, because _____

_____

12.   Have there been any short-term (five years or less) or long-term (five-, 10- or 15-year) studies of how patients do after this treatment?
❑ Yes ❑ No
If yes, do they evaluate:

- overall survival? (the chance of dying of any disease, especially prostate cancer, after treatment) ❑ Yes ❑ No
- disease-free survival? (the chance of dying only of prostate cancer after treatment) ❑ Yes ❑ No
- progression-free survival? (the chance of cancer advancing to another stage after treatment) ❑ Yes ❑ No
- metastasis rate? (the chance of cancer spreading to the bone or other organs after treatment) ❑ Yes ❑ No
- PSA changes over time? ❑ Yes ❑ No

13.   What kind of results can a man with my PSA level _____ grade _____ and stage _____ of cancer expect from this procedure? _____

_____

_____

14.   Can I talk to a patient who has had this treatment? (If your doctor is unable to locate a person who's willing to talk about his treatment experiences, you may have better luck through a local or national support group.) NOTE: Even if your doctor provides a list of patients who are willing to talk about their treatment, it is important also to contact patients who are not on that list. This helps ensure that the information is as unbiased as possible.

All treatments, drugs and diagnostic tests are considered experimental unless they are approved by an arm of the government called the U.S. Food and Drug Administration, or FDA. The FDA appoints temporary advisory committees to advise an FDA drug review group. Members of these advisory committees come from medical institutions, professional schools, government agencies, industry and trade associations, and consumer and patient groups nationwide.*

The FDA approval process takes a long time, in some cases up to 20 years, because federal regulators require that a drug undergo rigorous testing and evaluation to ensure that it is safe and effective (see Fig. 7A). In the late 1980s, however, the FDA introduced a faster approval system, but only for drugs or treatments that are used to treat life-threatening diseases. For example, under the older system, it took 21 years to approve Taxol, a drug for ovarian cancer. Under the faster system, it took only five years to approve an AIDS drug called DDC.

When a procedure is not FDA approved it could mean one of the following:

- Not enough information or research is yet known about the procedure to determine whether it is effective and safe.
- The procedure is safe and effective but has yet to be approved by the FDA because it takes time to get approval.
- The procedure is not safe and effective but has yet to be disapproved by the FDA because this, too, takes time.

FAST FACT

The FDA applies the same standards to over-the-counter, or OTC, medications as it does to prescription drugs. Since 1990 the FDA has banned at least 500 ingredients used for OTCs because of their lack of effectiveness.

---

* For information about FDA advisory committee meetings, call (800) 741-8138. In the Washington, D.C., area call (301) 443-0572. For information on how to nominate a consumer representative to an FDA advisory committee, write to the Office of Consumer Affairs, Food and Drug Administration, HFE-88, Room 16-85, 5600 Fishers Lane, Rockville, Md. 20857.

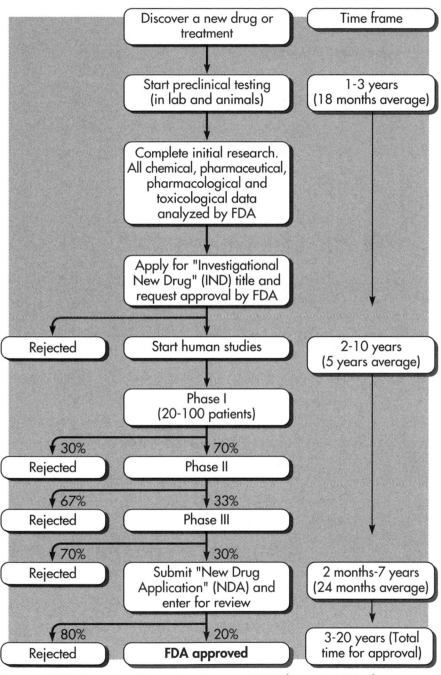

Source: *FDA Consumer Magazine*, January 1995 (second edition)

Fig. 7A — The Process for Achieving FDA Approval

When an investigational new drug is approved, human studies may begin.

B

Does 'freezing' the prostate really stop the cancer from spreading?

You may have heard on TV or read in the newspaper about a procedure called "prostatic cryoablation." This is just a medical term for freezing the prostate. The prefix "cryo" means "to freeze," and the word "ablation" means "to get rid of." So, prostatic cryoablation means to get rid of the prostate cancer by freezing it. Also called cryotherapy or cryosurgery, this is an experimental treatment that is NOT FDA APPROVED. It has probably not yet gained FDA approval because the treatment has undergone recent advances and not enough information is known about it. However, it is still a unique approach for treating prostate cancer that merits mention (see Table 7B).

How cryotherapy is performed

The night before the procedure an enema is given to clean out the rectal area, and antibiotics must be taken to decrease the chances of developing an infection.

During this transrectal ultrasound-guided procedure (performed under general or regional anesthesia), very cold liquid nitrogen (the same kind used in fire extinguishers) is used to freeze the prostate. Five small punctures are made in the perineum (the area between the testicles and anus), through which five metallic probes, or rods, are inserted. Liquid nitrogen is delivered through these rods into the prostate. The five thin metallic probes, each roughly 6 inches long, deliver temperatures of minus 185 to 195 degrees Celsius into the prostate until it becomes, quite literally, an "iceball" (see Fig. 7B).

Afterward, the frozen cancerous area melts; as it thaws, the cancer cells break apart, or burst. Although the prostate itself is frozen, the urethra (the urinary tract that runs through the gland) is kept warm during the procedure with a special warming device so that it is not damaged.

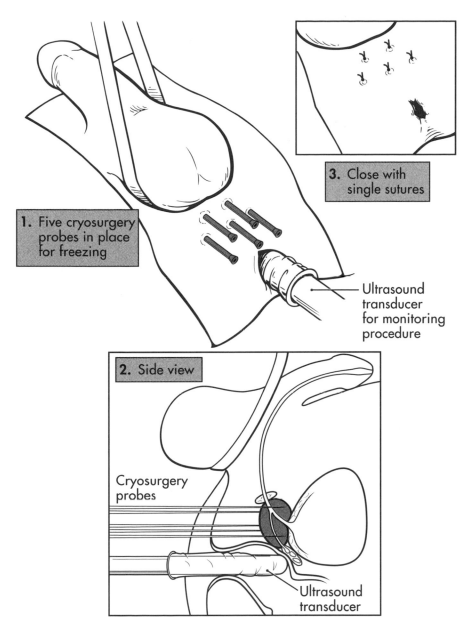

3. Close with single sutures

1. Five cryosurgery probes in place for freezing

Ultrasound transducer for monitoring procedure

2. Side view

Cryosurgery probes

Ultrasound transducer

Fig. 7B — Cryosurgery

During cryosurgery, five supercooled probes are inserted through the per-ineum (the area between the anus and scrotum) into different areas of the prostate. A transrectal ultrasound probe (covered with a condom) is insert-ed into the rectum to help guide the procedure. Top left: A frontal view. Bot-tom: A side view of the procedure. Top right: When the probes are removed, each of the punctures requires only a single suture, or stitch, to close.

Cryotherapy takes two to three hours. You either go home that day or stay overnight in the hospital. You will be given Motrin for any discomfort, and Hytrin or Cardura (medications that relax the prostate) to help reduce swelling for several weeks after the procedure. You will also continue to be on antibiotics for several days after the procedure, and a catheter and/or abdominal tube (called a suprapubic tube) must be used for two to three weeks until the swelling goes down and normal urination returns.

After the procedure, you will be monitored by PSA testing every three months. If your PSA levels begin to rise, a prostate biopsy may be performed to determine if there is residual cancer in the gland.

In the event of a positive biopsy, you could undergo cryoablation once again. Or, if you prefer, radical prostatectomy or external-beam radiation therapy could be used if the cancer is still confined to the prostate. You can begin normal activities about one to two weeks after the procedure.

Table 7B — **Report Card:** *Cryotherapy*

✔ **Effectiveness**	
Risk of cancer recurrence within six to 24 months	20-25%
Number of patients with a PSA level below 0.5 ng/ml after six months	80%
✔ **Side effects**	
Risk of impotence	90%
Risk of urethral blockage requiring surgical repair	25%
Risk of incontinence	5-15%
Risk of short-term penile numbness (Lasting less than six months)	10%
Risk of long-term perineal pain and ulceration	<5%
✔ **Total average cost**	$13,000–$15,000
(Not usually covered by insurance)	

The best candidates for cryotherapy are:

- older men (age 70 or above) with stage T1, T2 or T3 (A, B or C) prostate cancer;
- those who don't qualify for surgery or radiation therapy;
- those who don't want surgery or radiation therapy; and
- those who have failed radiation therapy.

The advantages of cryotherapy:

- It only requires a short hospital stay, if any.
- It is a relatively noninvasive procedure.

The disadvantages of cryotherapy:

- Impotence. About nine out of 10 patients (90 percent) experience long-term difficulties in having erections.
- Short-term urinary problems. Most patients will have problems urinating for several weeks after the procedure because the prostate enlarges temporarily and presses on the urethra, or urinary tract, cutting off flow.
- The long-term effectiveness and side effects of this procedure are not known.
- Cryosurgery is expensive. The total average cost is $13,000-$15,000, and many insurance companies do not cover the cost.

FAST FACT

The first cryosurgeries were performed in the 1960s.

C

What are radioactive-seed implants?

In the last chapter we talked about a type of radiation treatment called external-beam radiation therapy, in which radiation, delivered from an outside source, enters the body and targets the prostate in an attempt to kill the cancer cells. There is another treatment that uses radiation to fight prostate cancer, but this treatment uses many small "seeds" (each about the size of a grain of rice) of radioactive material that are implanted directly into the prostate gland. This procedure, called radioactive-seed implantation, has also been given a few fancy medical names: "interstitial brachytherapy," "brachytherapy" and "internal radiation."

The radioactive seeds (usually either Iodine 125 or Palladium 103) are placed inside the prostate tissue, hence the word "interstitial," which means "situated within." The prefix "brachy-" in medicine means "short," so the concept is to place the radioactive seeds within the prostate a short distance from the cancer, where it should be most effective in fighting it. The general idea is that radiation is delivered directly inside the prostate as opposed to traveling from the outside in. Some types of seeds remain permanently in place, while others are later removed.

Before the seeds are placed in the prostate, a great deal of time is spent understanding exactly where the cancer is and the precise location of the prostate. The idea here is that doctors want to know exactly where to place the radioactive seeds and how much radiation the seeds should give off. This will vary from patient to patient because the location and aggressiveness of a cancer can be different from one person to the next. In general, the higher the grade of cancer, the higher the dose of radiation, or isotope, is used. Iodine 125 seeds may be best for slow-growing, low-grade cancers, while Palladium 103 and the temporary seed implant Iridium 192 may be best for faster-growing, high-grade cancers. The higher the radiation dosage, the more effective the treatment — but the greater the severity of side effects (see Table 7C).

For at least 10 days before the procedure, you must stop using blood-thinning products such as aspirin to prevent excess bleeding. The night before, an enema must be used to empty the rectum, and no food or liquids are allowed until the procedure is over.

Permanent radioactive-seed implantation — Once the exact location of the prostate is determined through X-ray or ultrasound, between 70 and 150 seeds are implanted throughout the prostate via thin needles passed through the skin of the perineum (the area between the testicles and the anus). (See Fig. 7C-1.) The number of seeds used depends on the size of the prostate. An ultrasound probe is inserted into the rectum to help the surgeon determine the proper placement of the seeds. Initially, brachytherapy involved the use of low-dose seeds (Iodine 125), which were inserted into the prostate retropubically (via the abdomen) instead of the newer

---

Table 7C — **Report Card:** *Permanent Seed Implants*

✔ **Effectiveness**

Patients who are disease-free (based on PSA) five years after undergoing the older retropubic approach	74%
Patients who are disease-free (based on PSA) 10 years after undergoing the older retropubic approach	66%
(Long-term results of newer transperineal method are not available.)	

✔ **Side effects**

Within the first year

Risk of incontinence (with prior TURP)	6-29%
Risk of incontinence (without prior TURP)	0
Risk of proctitis, bloody stool, cystitis or bloody urine	85%

After the first year

Risk of partial impotence	20-30%
Risk of total impotence	20-30%
Risk of proctitis (rectal inflammation)	6-12%

✔ **Total average cost** | $15,000-
(Not covered by insurance) | $25,000

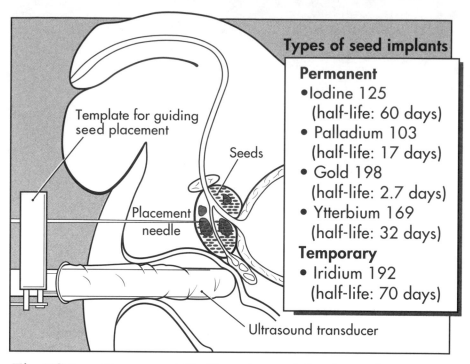

Types of seed implants

Permanent
- Iodine 125
  (half-life: 60 days)
- Palladium 103
  (half-life: 17 days)
- Gold 198
  (half-life: 2.7 days)
- Ytterbium 169
  (half-life: 32 days)

Temporary
- Iridium 192
  (half-life: 70 days)

Fig. 7C-1 — Permanent Radioactive-seed Implantation

A side view of permanent radioactive-seed implantation performed under the guidance of transrectal ultrasound, or TRUS. Small box: the various types of radioactive seeds used, the most popular of which are Palladium 103 and Iodine 125.

Note:

Today, most men who receive seed implants also undergo external-beam radiation either before or after this procedure to boost its overall effectiveness.

transperineal approach. This technique was more invasive and less accurate than the type of seed implantation performed today.

The procedure itself, performed under spinal anesthesia, lasts about 45 minutes to an hour, after which a catheter is placed until the numbness wears off — about two hours. Once the catheter is removed you can go home. Driving is prohibited for the first 12 hours, and strenuous activity should be avoided for 48 hours. After two to three days, normal activities can be resumed. And although this type of radiation probably does not escape the prostate, for the first couple of months it is recommended that those with implants should stay at least 6 feet away from pregnant women and children, who are most sensitive to radiation. The radioactivity itself is usually gone after one year.

The best candidates for permanent radioactive-seed implantation are:
- men with localized prostate cancer (stages T1 or T2; A or B) who have a life expectancy of at least 10 years;
- older men (70 and above) with localized prostate cancer who are not candidates for surgery due to other medical conditions; and
- some men with locally advanced prostate cancer (stage T3 or C).

Advantages of permanent seed implantation:
- Results indicate that it is as effective as external beam radiation or surgery in the short term (up to five years).
- In some cases there is no need for additional external-beam radiation therapy.
- Seed implants deliver about twice the effective dose of radiation to the prostate vs. that of external-beam radiation alone.
- The procedure is relatively noninvasive.
- There is minimal affect on urinary control and minimal associated bleeding.
- It is a new technique, so its effectiveness may continue to improve.
- It is covered by Medicare and other forms of insurance.

Disadvantages of permanent seed implantation:
- Long-term (10- and 15-year) results of the newer and more effective transperineal procedure, combined with external-beam radiation, are not yet available.
- Most long-term data collected to date are from one institution.
- It is not FDA approved.

- Its complications include difficulty urinating, rectal discomfort, sexual dysfunction and swelling or inflammation of the prostate.
- After undergoing this procedure, a man is usually no longer a candidate for surgery.
- It is expensive, with a total average cost of $15,000 to $25,000.

Temporary radioactive-seed implantation — This procedure, also called "iridium template therapy," "high-dose-rate (HDR) brachytherapy," and "fractionated HDR conformal prostate brachytherapy" is a little different from the standard ultrasound-guided permanent seed implant procedure. It involves placing an intense radiation source directly into or around the cancer for a short period of time (see Fig. 7C-2). After the patient receives a spinal anesthetic, 12-20 small, flexible plastic needles are inserted through the perineum and into the prostate. This is done under ultrasound guidance, and the procedure itself takes about one and

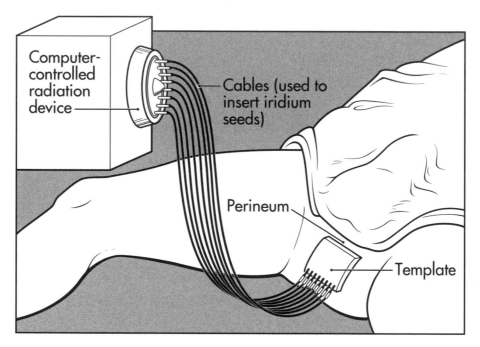

Fig. 7C-2— Temporary Radioactive -seed Implantation

Iridium seeds (also called "bars") are inserted and timed using a computer-controlled radiation device.

a half hours. A small plastic plate, which holds the needles in place, is left next to the perineum. A bladder catheter inserted during the procedure is also kept in place until the next day.

Radiation treatment planning, based on a CT scan of the prostate, begins after the needles are inserted. After the strategy is approved, the patient receives the first of three high-dose-radiation (HDR) treatments. An HDR machine under computer control transfers an intense radioactive source to each implanted needle. The treatment takes five to eight minutes and is painless. The remaining two treatments are given the next day, in the morning and afternoon. After the last HDR treatment, the template, needles and bladder catheter are removed. Once the patient is able to urinate, he is able to leave the hospital. The patient should spend a quiet evening at home and the next day a radiation oncologist or urologist will meet with the patient to examine the perineum.

The second phase of treatment involves external-beam radiation therapy (usually about two weeks later). This typically involves 20 individual external-beam radiation treatments given daily, Monday through Friday, for four weeks.

The short-term side effects of temporary seed implants include:
- urinary frequency and burning
- rectal irritation
- intestinal gas
- soft bowel movements
- mild fatigue

Advantages of temporary seed implants:
- Between 60 percent and 80 percent of those who are fully potent before the procedure will remain potent afterward. Any symptoms of impotence are usually temporary.
- Most men continue to work full time during the follow-up external-beam radiation therapy.
- The three-year disease-free survival rate is 85 percent.

Disadvantages of temporary seed implants:

- About 5 percent of patients experience minor urethral strictures (narrowing of the urethra with scar tissue), which may require treatment.
- Patients who have had a previous transurethral resection of the prostate, or TURP, usually don't qualify for the procedure.
- The procedure is expensive, costing about 35 percent to 50 percent more than a standard ultrasound-guided seed-implant procedure.
- This is a very new procedure, so there are no long-term data on its effectiveness.

To summarize: the complication rate, time involved, pain and dollar cost is lower with the permanent seed implant procedure vs. that of the temporary iridium template procedure. However, early results suggest that it may be as effective as permanent seed implantation.

FAST FACT

The first research results on brachytherapy (radioactive-seed implantation) for prostate cancer were published in 1911.

The ABCs of CHAPTER 7
A Quick Review

A

How do I decide if an experimental approach may be right for me?

- When considering an experimental therapy — or any treatment, for that matter — get a general description of the treatment, for whom the treatment is best suited, and its advantages and disadvantages. Then, bring a list of more specific questions to your doctor or support group.

- If your prostate cancer is localized (confined to the prostate) then ask how this treatment compares to the two most effective treatments today — radical prostatectomy and external-beam radiation therapy.

- If your prostate cancer has spread beyond the prostate, then ask how it compares to external-beam radiation therapy, the most commonly used treatment for locally advanced cancer (cancer that has invaded neighboring tissues).

B

Does 'freezing' the prostate really stop the cancer from spreading?

- Men who qualify for cryoablation include those who have failed radiation therapy, those whose cancer has spread just beyond the prostate, those over age 70 and men with confined or localized disease who do not want surgery or radiation.

- The advantages of freezing the prostate include a short hospital stay, few short-term side effects, and the fact that it is less invasive than surgery and is easily done.

- The disadvantages of freezing the prostate include a high incidence of impotence (about nine out of 10 patients), and temporary urinary difficulty. Also, it is not FDA approved and in some states this $13,000-$15,000 procedure is not covered by insurance.

C

What are radioactive-seed implants?

- Seed implants, also known as interstitial brachytherapy, are a method of delivering radiation internally to kill cancer cells.
- To qualify for this procedure, a man may have localized, organ-confined or locally advanced (C or T3) prostate cancer.
- While seed implants are relatively noninvasive, there are no long-term data on the effectiveness of the newer transperineal technique. However, five-year data suggests that they are as effective as external-beam radiation therapy and radical prostatectomy in the short term.

- Complications of seed implants include rectal and sexual problems and inflammation of the prostate.
- Iridium template therapy, or high-dose-rate (HDR) brachytherapy (also called "fractionated HDR conformal prostate brachytherapy"), involves placing a temporary intense radiation source directly into or around the cancer for a short period of time. After these temporary iridium seeds are removed, the patient undergoes external-beam radiation therapy. The complication rate, time involved, pain and dollar cost is lower with the permanent seed implant procedure vs. this temporary seed implantation technique. However, early results suggest that it may be as effective as permanent seed implantation.

Medical References

Title: **"Cryosurgical ablation of the prostate: two-year prostate-specific antigen and biopsy results"**
Authors: Cohen, J.K.; Miller, R.J.; Rooker, G.M.; et al
Journal: *Urology*
Volume: 47 (3)
Pages: 395-401
Date: March 1996

Title: **"Does brachytherapy have a role in the treatment of prostate cancer"**
Authors: Grimm, P.D.; Blasko, J.C.; Ragde, H.; et al
Journal: *Hematology/Oncology Clinics of North America*
Volume: 10 (3)
Pages: 653-673
Date: June 1996

Title: **"Complications of cryosurgical ablation of the prostate to treat localized adenocarcinoma of the prostate"**
Authors: Cox, R.L.; and Crawford, E.D.
Journal: *Urology*
Volume: 45 (6)
Pages: 932-935
Date: June 1995

Title: **"Prostate Cancer Clinical Guidelines Panel summary report on management of clinically localized prostate cancer"**
Authors: Middleton, R.D.; Thompson, I.M.; Austenfield, M.S.; et al
Journal: *Journal of Urology*
Volume: 154
Pages: 2144-2148
Date: December 1995

Title: **"Brachytherapy for prostate cancer"**
Authors: Porter, A.T.; Blasko, J.C.; Grimm, P.D.; et al
Journal: *CA — Cancer Journal for Clinicians*
Volume: 45 (3)
Pages: 165-178
Date: May-June 1995

Notes _____

_____

_____

_____

_____

_____

_____

_____

_____

_____

_____

_____

_____

_____

_____

_____

_____

_____

_____

8

The Cancer Has Spread Beyond the Prostate:

How Hormonal Therapy Can Help

A

What is single-agent androgen-deprivation (hormonal) therapy?

B

What is combination androgen-deprivation (complete hormonal) therapy?
What is the latest word on chemotherapy?

C

What are the best strategies for dealing with cancer pain?

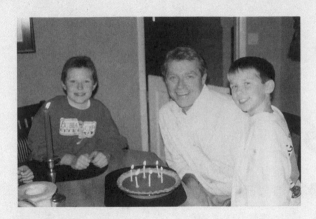

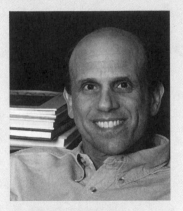

Jerry VerDorn
Actor ('Guiding Light')

I found out I had cancer at age 43 through the PSA blood test. My prostate felt perfectly normal, so a digital-rectal exam alone would not have found it. A blood test that can tell you so much is a gift — all men should take advantage of it.

For the first week of my radiation therapy, I would just lie there for about 10 minutes, alone in the room with this big machine, and find myself weeping and thinking, "This can't be happening." And then I got over that and started trying to help the machine through positive mental imaging. I got very much into alternative medicine and that helped me a lot, because it gave me something active to do instead of just having people and machines do things to me. I think this way, the doctor had a better patient on his hands too; someone who was willing to fight instead of being just a lump lying there.

Basically, my advice to those who've been recently diagnosed with prostate cancer is: Don't be afraid to get angry and go through the "why me" phase. Once you go through that, if you're at all resilient, you'll get tired of thinking that way and you'll suddenly look at the universe and say, "Well, why not me?" And then, "What am I going to do about it?" You can gather your friends and family around you, and you can gather information about the disease; those are the two things that are going to help get you through it.

Jerry VerDorn with his sons Jacob, 13, (left) and Peter, 11, above.

Michael Milken
Founder, chairman and
president of CaP Cure

In January 1993, I had a routine physical and requested a PSA test, even though I was only 46 years old. Everything was fine, except that my PSA came back with a score of 24. To say the news was devastating would be a gross understatement.

I had planned on having a prostatectomy, but further tests found that my lymph nodes had been affected by the cancer, so removing the gland wouldn't serve a purpose. I was stunned. The good news was that the cancer had not spread to my bones. My doctors then prescribed hormone therapy and radiation treatment to slow the cancer growth, and my PSA eventually dropped from 24 to 0, where it remains today. Even though my cancer can be considered advanced, I have never experienced a symptom – no bone pain, no fatigue and no weight loss. That's what's so frightening about this disease.

I am optimistic that future research will provide more effective treatments and a cure for prostate cancer. The technology, basic science and creative minds are there, but the financial support is lacking. This gap can be closed by writing or calling your political representatives to increase funds for cancer research. The potential benefits are immeasurable.

A

What is single-agent androgen-deprivation (hormonal) therapy?

Before discussing the different types of hormonal therapy used to treat advanced prostate cancer, it is important to understand the various stages of prostate-cancer growth:

Locally advanced — When the malignancy has spread to neighboring tissues such as the seminal vesicles (stage C or T3) or involves other pelvic organs, such as the rectum or bladder (stage C, D or T4).

Regionally advanced — When the cancer has spread to the lymph nodes (stage D1+ or N+).

Advanced, or metastatic — When the cancer has spread to the bones (stage D2+ or M+).

More general terms used to describe cancer that has spread beyond the prostate include "not confined" and "not localized."

Regardless of what advanced prostate cancer is called, there are many options that must be carefully examined and discussed with the doctor before choosing the right treatment. The most common type of treatment for advanced prostate cancer is called single-agent androgen-deprivation therapy, or hormonal therapy (also called partial hormonal therapy, or monotherapy). ("Androgen" is just a fancy name for male hormones; "deprivation" refers to depriving the body of these hormones by blocking their production and/or action. "Single agent" means that a single procedure or drug is used to accomplish this task.)

It is important to remember that such therapy, also called palliative treatment, is not usually a cure, but it can increase the length and quality of your life.

Certain male hormones, or androgens, promote the growth of prostate cancer, much like throwing gasoline (hormones) on a fire (cancer). Single-agent androgen-deprivation therapy puts that fire out by interrupting the pathway of hormone production that speeds the growth of cancer cells.

Cancer cells that grow faster and do more damage when hormones are present are called "hormone-sensitive cancer cells." Cancer cells that grow at a pace that is unaffected by hormones are called "hormone-insensitive cancer cells." Prostate cancer consists of both types of cells, and every man's ratio of sensitive to insensitive cells is different. The more hormone-sensitive cells you have, the better you'll respond to hormone therapy. The more hormone-insensitive cells you have, the less successful your results will be from such treatment.

Today there is not a great deal we can do about the hormone-insensitive cells, but with the current pace of prostate-cancer research, this may soon change. We can, however, do something about the hormone-sensitive prostate cancer cells, and that is to cut off their fuel supply, or the amount of male hormone these cells receive. One hormone that can really fuel the prostate-cancer fire is testosterone, which is made mostly in the testicles. The testicles are located inside the scrotum, the pouch of skin below the penis.

Bilateral orchiectomy (surgical castration)

One way to decrease the body's testosterone level is to remove the testicles in a surgical procedure called bilateral orchiectomy. The word "bilateral" refers to "both" (in this case both testicles), the prefix "orchi-" means "testicles," and the suffix "-ectomy" means "the removal of." Basically, it just a fancy medical term for castration. Only the testicles themselves are removed, not the scrotum. The spermatic cord is also left, which helps retain the natural appearance of the scrotum (see Fig. 8A-1). To ensure an even more natural look, an artificial testicular implant can be placed in the scrotum during the testicle-removal surgery.

The best candidates for bilateral orchiectomy are (see Table 8A-1):

- asymptomatic or symptomatic men with locally advanced prostate cancer (stages C or T3) or cancer that has spread to other parts of the body (stages D, T3, T4, N + or M +).

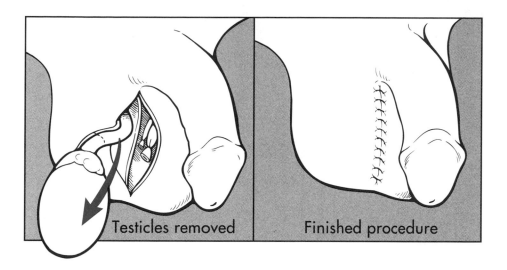

Testicles removed | Finished procedure

Fig. 8A-1 — Bilateral Orchiectomy (Surgical Hormonal Therapy)

Left: an incision is made between the two scrotal sacs and each testicle is removed from its spermatic cord. Right: The incision is then closed and the scrotum retains its normal appearance.

Advantages of bilateral orchiectomy:

- It is easy and inexpensive (as compared with the other treatment options for advanced prostate cancer).
- It can be done on an outpatient basis.
- Even though the testicles are removed, the scrotum remains, which maintains a normal appearance.
- It is very effective in reducing the amount of testosterone in the body.
- Its impact is immediate: almost all of the body's testosterone is gone within hours after the surgery, and there is no chance of it returning because its main production source has been eliminated. The smaller amount of testosterone that remains (5 percent to 10 percent) comes from the adrenal glands, which are located on top of the kidneys.
- Perhaps most important, although castration is a permanent procedure that cannot be reversed, it can increase the quality and quantity of one's life.

Table 8A-1 — **Report Card:** *Bilateral Orchiectomy*

✔ **Effectiveness**

Survival rate (locally advanced — stages T3 and T4):

Five-year	50-60%
Ten-year	40%

Survival rate (metastatic — stages D1 and D2):

Two-year	50%
Five-year	20-30%

Effectiveness in decreasing bone pain	75%
Effectiveness in decreasing PSA levels	75%

✔ **Side effects**

Risk of decreased sex drive	almost 100%
Risk of impotence	almost 100%
Risk of hot flashes	50%
Risk of breast enlargement, nipple sensitivity	50%
Risk of weight gain	90%

✔ **Total average cost** $2,000-$4,000
(Covered by most insurance,
including Medicaid)

Disadvantages of bilateral orchiectomy:

- It causes decreased sex drive, or libido, in most men.
- It causes erectile dysfunction (the decreased ability to have an erection) or impotence in most men.
- It is unable to eliminate the small amount (5 percent to 10 percent) of testosterone produced by the adrenal glands that continues to circulate in the body.
- It causes hot flashes, similar to those that women get during menopause, in about half of those who undergo the procedure. However, there are a number of medications that can treat these symptoms, such as estrogen, megace, Provera and clonidine.
- It causes slight breast enlargement (also called gynecomastia) and nipple tenderness or sensitivity in about half of those who have the surgery.

- It causes weight gain around the midsection (between 10 and 15 pounds).

- It is not reversible. Once the testicles are removed, they cannot be replaced.

- Another concern is psychological; feeling a loss of manhood. There is nothing we can say in a few sentences to prevent men from feeling this possible loss, but it is important to focus on the fact that one's life is being preserved and prolonged.

LHRH agonists

There are some very good nonsurgical alternatives to bilateral orchiectomy. The first is a form of single-agent hormonal therapy that uses a class of drugs called "LHRH agonists."

LHRH is a protein produced deep in the brain that stimulates the production of something called leutenizing hormone, or LH, which in turn increases the production of testosterone. An LHRH agonist is a synthetic hormone, similar in structure to the brain's natural LHRH, which when injected into the patient eventually turns off the production of LH and therefore halts testosterone production.

Some of the commonly prescribed LHRH agonists include leupro- lide acetate (Lupron), made by Abbott Laboratories; and goserelin acetate (Zoladex), made by Zeneca Pharmaceuticals.

These medications are given by an injection in the hip once a month for the rest of your life (unless you choose later to have a bilateral orchiectomy). However, there are new, stronger forms of Lupron and Zoladex that only need to be given once every three months (see Fig. 8A-2). So instead of going to the doctor for an injection every month, you now only need to go four times a year.

The first time an LHRH agonist is injected, it temporarily increas- es testosterone production for the first seven to 10 days. This brief surge in testosterone can cause a condition called "tumor flare" in about 10 percent to 30 percent of patients, in which symptoms tem- porarily become worse. However an antiandrogen medication can be given at the same time to prevent the initial testosterone spike (also see Chapter 7, Section B). After the first week to 10 days, the

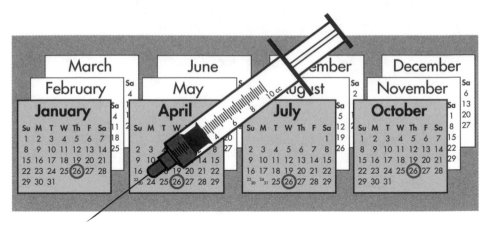

Fig. 8A-2 — LHRH Agonist Injections (Medical Hormonal Therapy)

LHRH agonist injections only need to be given once every three months, in a doctor's office.

drug starts working to shut off the testosterone supply. Therefore, the eventual effect is similar to a bilateral orchiectomy in that the body's testosterone level drops to near zero (see Table 8A-2).

The best candidates for LHRH agonists are:

• asymptomatic or symptomatic men with locally advanced prostate cancer (stages C, T3 or T4) or cancer that has spread to other parts of the body (stages D, T3, T4, N+ or M+).

Advantages of LHRH agonists:

• They are as effective as testicle-removal surgery in decreasing testosterone levels to near zero.

• They are as effective as surgery in increasing the quality and quantity of life.

• Testicle-removal surgery can still be an option later on.

Disadvantages of LHRH agonists:

• They cause decreased libido, or sex drive, in most men.

• They cause erectile dysfunction or impotence in most men.

• They may require the additional use of an antiandrogen medication at the beginning of treatment to prevent tumor flare.

Table 8A-2 — **Report Card:** *LHRH Agonists*

✔ **Effectiveness**

Survival rate (locally advanced — stages T3 and T4):	
Five-year	50-60%
Ten-year	40%
Survival rate (metastatic — stages D1 and D2):	
Two-year	50%
Five-year	20-30%

✔ **Side effects**

Risk of decreased sex drive	almost 100%
Risk of impotence	almost 100%
Risk of hot flashes	50% (60-65% with three-month injections)
Risk of breast enlargement and nipple sensitivity	50-70%
Risk of weight gain	90%
Risk of tumor flare if taken without an antiandrogen	8-32%

✔ **Total average cost** $4,000–$6,000 a year

- They cause hot flashes similar to those experienced by women during menopause. However, there are a number of medications that can treat this uncomfortable symptom.

- They cause slight breast enlargement and nipple tenderness or sensitivity in about half of the men who take them. However, this can be prevented with several low-dosage radiation treatments to the breast (also can be done with bilateral orchiectomy patients).

- They cause weight gain around the midsection (between 10 and 15 pounds) in most men.

- They require regular trips to the doctor for injections for the rest of the patient's life.

- They can cause the testicles to decrease in size.

- The injections are expensive, about $4,000-$6,000 a year.

Estrogen therapy

There are also a number of single-agent therapies that are mostly derived from estrogen, the female hormone, which can serve as an alternative to surgery (bilateral orchiectomy) and LHRH-agonist therapy. They include:

DES — This stands for diethylstilbestrol, an estrogen that stops the production of testosterone. For effectiveness in reducing testosterone and its side effects, DES is the clear choice if you are considering an estrogen medication (see Table 8A-3). However, it takes about two weeks before DES can coax the testosterone level down to near zero, so it is not as fast-acting as testicle-removal surgery or LHRH agonists. It is, however, as effective as surgery in enhancing the length and quality of life.

Table 8A-3 — **Report Card:** *DES (Estrogen Therapy)*

✔ **Effectiveness**

Survival rate (locally advanced — stages T3 and T4):

Five-year	50-60 %
Ten-year	40 %

Survival rate (metastatic — stages D1 and D2):

Two-year	50 %
Five-year	20-30 %

✔ **Side effects**

Risk of decreased sex drive	almost 100 %
Risk of impotence	almost 100 %
Risk of breast enlargement and nipple sensitivity	50-70 %
Risk of weight gain	90 %

✔ **Total average cost** — $100–$500 a year

There is some controversy regarding the optimum daily dosage of DES, which is taken in pill form. The greater the amount of DES given the better it lowers testosterone, but the potential for side effects such as heart disease, stroke and blood clots also increases. Research has shown that 3 mg (milligrams) of DES daily may be the right amount, because it is enough to lower testosterone levels without causing heart disease and other serious side effects. Some doctors prefer to give a higher dosage than 3 mg, but again, that carries a greater risk for dangerous side effects. In addition, research has shown that 3 mg of DES daily increases the life span as effectively as higher dosages. Current research is investigating the possibility of combining DES with an antiandrogen for more effective results.

The best candidates for DES are:

- asymptomatic or symptomatic men with locally advanced prostate cancer (stages C, T3 or T4) or cancer that has spread to other parts of the body (stages D, T3, T4, N+ and M+).

Advantages of DES:

- It is as effective as a bilateral orchiectomy or LHRH agonists in reducing testosterone production.
- Since it is in pill form, it does not require regular doctor visits to be taken, as with LHRH-agonist injections.
- It is inexpensive ($100-$500 a year).
- It does not limit the use of other treatments down the road, such as bilateral orchiectomy or other forms of hormonal therapy.

Disadvantages of DES:

- It takes about two weeks before testosterone levels begin to drop.
- It carries the risk of side effects such as heart disease. In addition to keeping the daily dose low, at 3 mg, some doctors have their patients take an aspirin each day to further reduce their cardiac risk. However, anyone with cardiovascular problems or problems with clotting in the legs (also called thrombophlebitis) should not use any estrogen-derived medications.
- It causes decreased libido, or sex drive, in most men.

- It causes erectile dysfunction, or impotence, in most men.
- It causes breast enlargement, which can be prevented with several low-dosage radiation treatments to the breast before estrogen therapy begins.
- It causes swelling (also called edema) in certain areas such as the ankles and feet, which can be treated with diuretics, medications that cause a person to shed excess water by urinating more often.
- It must be taken daily for the rest of the man's life.

Other estrogen-derived therapies

The following medications can be as effective as DES but should be considered only if DES is not working or cannot be taken:

EMCYT (estramustine phosphate) — this drug has shown some success in Europe, but it can cause side effects such as nausea and vomiting.

Ethinyl estradiol and Premarin — These are taken orally and are also used by women during menopause.

Esradurin — This is injected once a month. A good choice for patients with stomach or digestive problems.

Stilphostrol — This is given daily via injection. This is an excellent estrogen therapy for immediately decreasing testosterone levels.

FAST FACT

About three out of every 10 men (30 percent) with prostate cancer have used LHRH agonists. About one out of every 10 men (10 percent) with prostate cancer have had a bilateral orchiectomy (castration).

B

What is combination androgen-deprivation (complete hormonal) therapy?

In single-agent androgen-deprivation therapy, one drug or one procedure causes a dramatic decrease in a certain type of androgen, or male hormone — usually testosterone that is produced by the testicles. However, research has shown that up to 10 percent of the total hormone levels within the prostate can come from the adrenal glands. Combination androgen-deprivation therapy (also called combined hormonal therapy, or CHT; or maximal androgen blockade) pairs an LHRH agonist or bilateral orchiectomy with something called an "antiandrogen" drug to shut down this additional source of testosterone production, as well as the production of other types of male hormones that fuel prostate cancer (see Table 8B).

Table 8B — **Report Card:** *Antiandrogens Combined with LHRH Agonists*

✔ **Effectiveness**	
Survival rate (locally advanced — stages T3 and T4)	unknown
Survival rate (metastatic — stage D2)	
Two-year	60%
Five-year	30-40%
✔ **Side effects**	
Risk of decreased sex drive	almost 100%
Risk of impotence	almost 100%
Risk of hot flashes	more than 50%
Risk of breast enlargement and nipple sensitivity	50-70%
Risk of diarrhea/constipation	10-20%
Risk of nausea/vomiting	3-11%
✔ **Total average cost**	$6,000–$10,000 per year

An antiandrogen is a type of drug that allows testosterone and other male hormones, or androgens, to be made and travel through the body but prevents them from interacting with cancerous cells. Again, it is important to remember that for complete effectiveness, antiandrogens must be used in combination with an LHRH agonist or a bilateral orchiectomy. These drugs should not be taken alone.

The best candidates for antiandrogens (combined with LHRH agonists or bilateral orchiectomy) are:

- asymptomatic or symptomatic men with locally advanced prostate cancer (stages C, T3 or T4) or cancer that has spread to other parts of the body (stages D, T3, T4, N+ or M+).

Types of antiandrogens

Eulexin (flutamide) — Made by Schering-Plough Corp., this is one of the most common antiandrogens. It must be taken for the rest of the man's life. When taken alone, it does not decrease testosterone levels, so most men do not have a decrease in sexual drive and most men do not have a decrease in the ability to have a natural erection. However, it causes diarrhea in 15 percent to 25 percent of those who take it, and it can cause liver problems in up to 2 percent of patients. It also can cause breast enlargement and nipple sensitivity. Some patients must be taken off flutamide if their cancer begins to grow again and their PSA level increases. This is because in some cases when a cancer has changed or mutated, flutamide may actually encourage the cancer to grow. This is called "androgen withdrawal syndrome."

Casodex (bicalutamide) — Made by Zeneca Pharmaceuticals, this is another frequently prescribed antiandrogen that also must be taken for the duration of the man's life. Like flutamide, when taken alone it does not decrease the sex drive or erectile function because it does not interfere with testosterone production, nor does it cause significant diarrhea. However, like flutamide, it can cause breast enlargement and nipple sensitivity in the majority of patients who take it. The "androgen-withdrawal syndrome" also has been reported with Casodex.

Nilandron (nilutamide) — Made by Hoechst Marion Roussel, this is a new antiandrogen that has recently gained FDA approval.

This drug's effectiveness is similar to flutamide and bicalutamide. However, it can produce two additional side effects: interstitial pneumonitis (lung inflammation) and difficulty seeing in the dark. The incidence of lung inflammation is less than 2 percent; approximately 13 percent report difficulty seeing in the dark.

Cyproterone acetate — This is a less widely used antiandrogen that is not FDA approved. It decreases the supply of testosterone, which means most men will have problems with sexual drive and impotence when taking it.

Ketoconazole — This drug, approved by the FDA as an antifungal agent, is used in short-term, urgent situations to immediately lower testosterone levels and thus shrink tumors — to relieve pressure on the spinal cord caused by a tumor on the vertebral column, for example. When taken three times a day, it knocks testosterone levels down to almost zero within 24 hours. It not only blocks testosterone production in the testicles but it also blocks the small amount of testosterone produced by the adrenal glands, which sit on top of the kidneys. The drug may cause a testosterone increase in the long term, so it should be used only to achieve a quick drop in hormone levels. Also, this drug stops the production of steroids by the adrenal glands. Thus, a prescribed steroid medication should also be taken along with it. Finally, there have been some liver problems associated with this drug, so again, it should only be used in the short term.

Many studies have shown that patients on combination therapy live a few months longer than those on single-agent therapy. So the advantage of combination therapy is not great. However, for patients who have early advanced prostate cancer (cancer that escaped the prostate but has minimally spread throughout the body), survival can be increased by an average of seven months. So, earlier combination treatment may mean more effective combination treatment.

Finally, as a reminder, all types of androgen-deprivation (single-agent or combination) only work on the hormone-sensitive cancer cells. Eventually the hormone-insensitive cancer cells will com-

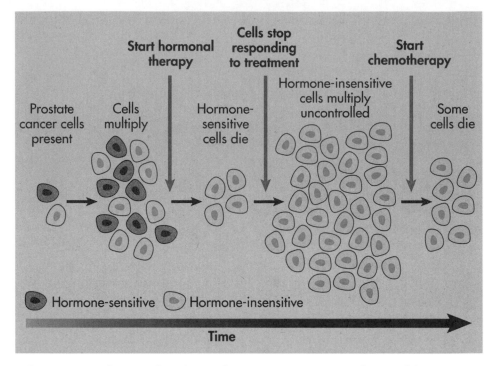

Fig. 8B — The Mechanism of Prostate-cancer Relapse (the Long-term Response of Cancer Cells to Hormonal Therapy and Chemotherapy)

Hormonal therapy kills hormone-sensitive cells, but eventually these cells are replaced by hormone-insensitive cells, which do not respond to hormonal treatment.

Chemotherapy, however, kills all types of cells — hormone-sensitive, hormone-insensitive, and normal prostate cells. Eventually, however, hormone-insensitive cells become resistant to chemotherapy, and thus multiply and spread out of control.

pletely take over, and that is why androgen deprivation is not a cure but a temporary treatment to help ease symptoms and extend a patient's life (see Fig. 8B).

Beyond hormonal therapy: chemotherapy

If hormonal therapy fails, as shown by a bone scan or a rising PSA level, then other drug treatments (chemotherapy) can be explored.

One such drug is suramin, which may be used to combat hormone-resistant cells and, at the same time, block androgen release from the adrenal glands. The drug's effectiveness is not known; it appears to work for some individuals but not others. When it does work, its benefit is only temporary. The potential side effects of suramin are serious: It can lower the body's immune system, which increases the risk of infections; it can decrease the body's blood-platelet count, which can interfere with blood clotting; and it can cause pain and fatigue.

The challenge in developing drug treatments for any type of cancer is that malignant tissue consists of cells that are "heterogeneous," or very different from each other. As mentioned earlier, when it comes to prostate cancer, there are basically two types of cancer cells: hormone-sensitive (responsive to hormone therapy) and hormone-insensitive (resistant to hormone therapy). However, even within those two groups of cells there are very large differences between them. Therefore, research has been focusing on a number of drugs that can be combined to battle the different kinds of cancer cells that co-exist. To this end, offshoots of many types of drugs, including suramin, are being combined and tested.

Traditionally, chemotherapy has done very little to extend the quantity or quality of life in men with prostate cancer. However, this may change because more and more institutions are trying some unique, experimental "combination chemotherapy" treatments in which several cancer-fighting drugs are used at once. For example, in recent animal studies, a combination of the drugs Estramustine, Etoposide and Taxol caused a greater than 90-percent decrease in cancer growth within two weeks. These drugs are now being tested in humans who are no longer responding to hormonal therapy — with promising initial results.

FAST FACT

Two out of every 10 men (20 percent) with advanced prostate cancer have received complete hormonal therapy, which is the combined use of castration or LHRH agonists with an antiandrogen drug.

C
What are the best strategies for dealing with cancer pain?

First and foremost, there is no need for a patient with advanced prostate cancer to experience a great deal of pain. Period. Cancer pain is generally divided into two categories: concentrated, or "spot," pain; and generalized, more widespread pain.

Spot pain

If an individual has pain in a specific area of the body (also called spot pain or concentrated pain) there are three very good treatment options:

Spot radiation — This is similar to external-beam radiation treatment, except that the radiation is targeted to the pain site, not necessarily to the cancer site (see Fig. 8C). The majority of patients (70 percent to 80 percent) who receive spot radiation experience complete or partial pain relief.

Strontium — This is actually called radioactive strontium 89, and it is effective in treating bone pain (see Table 8C). Once injected, this compound is absorbed by the bones. Cancerous bone actually absorbs strontium better than other tissues, so this may be why the majority of patients feel better after just one injection. The effect is long-lasting, so the drug can prevent pain caused by any additional cancer growth after the first injection. Strontium injections are given on the average of once every six months. They should not be given in intervals of less than 90 days.

The advantages of strontium:

- It is as effective and more easily tolerated than spot radiation treatment for cancer pain.
- It is easy and fast to administer.
- It works only in the cancerous areas.
- The patient is not a radiation hazard to others.

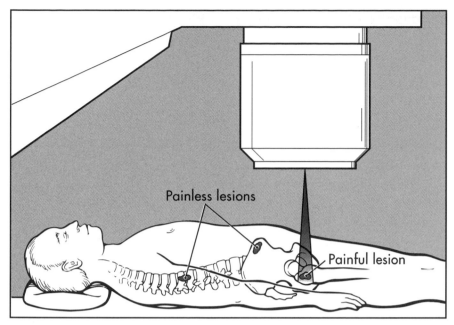

Fig. 8C — Spot-radiation Therapy

This pain-management technique targets external-beam radiation to the site of cancer pain, not necessarily to the cancer itself.

Table 8C — **Report Card:***Strontium 89*

✔ **Effectiveness**

Percentage of patients who experience partial or complete pain relief	80%
The average amount of time it takes to get partial or complete pain relief	10-20 days
The average length of time pain relief lasts after treatment	4-15 months
The percentage decrease in pain medication use after treatment	50%

✔ **Side effects**

The No. 1 side effect is blood disorders, but they usually don't require medical attention.	
The average decrease in platelet count after treatment	24-50%

✔ **Total average cost**

	$1,000-$2,000 (vs. $3,000-$4,000 for spot radiation)

The disadvantages of strontium:

- It can damage the bone marrow, which could cause a problem with blood clotting.

- It may cause short-term pain at the beginning of treatment, which is actually a good indicator of a better long-term result. The pain can be countered with other pain medications.

- Radioactive urine must be disposed in a special container for the first few days after injection.

Combination strontium/radiation therapy — The most effective treatment for specific pain seems to be a combination of strontium and spot radiation. Initial studies have shown that together they can keep pain at bay for several months longer than when used individually.

Generalized pain

There are so many medications that treat general body pain that we would need a number of pages just to list the ones available right now. If you are experiencing generalized pain, the best thing to do is to talk to your doctor about the kind of pain you are feeling.

Over-the-counter medications and prescription drugs — If your pain is as bothersome as, say, a mild headache, the doctor may suggest you try over-the-counter drugs such as acetaminophen (Tylenol) or ibuprofen (Motrin), or one of many prescription drugs for light pain. If the pain is constant and moderate or strong, then there are a number of possible narcotics that are effective, such as codeine and morphine. The key is to rate your pain (on a scale of one to 10, for example) so you'll be able to tell the doctor specifically how much pain you are experiencing.

Also, if you are worried about becoming addicted to narcotics, don't be. There is no evidence to show that these pain medications are addictive; in fact research has shown that pain management can increase the quality as well as the quantity of life.

Drug patches — There are also new ways pain medication can be delivered. One unique way that has gained some attention is through a patch that is placed on the body. The patch can help those with strong or severe pain by releasing pain medication through the skin on a regular basis. Tell your doctor what you are comfortable with and work together to not only choose the right medication but the way you would like it administered.

Wide-field radiation — Also called "hemibody" radiation, this technique for managing generalized pain involves the use of radiation throughout the body.

Advantages of wide-field radiation:

- About half of patients who undergo hemibody radiation experience partial or complete pain relief within 48 hours of treatment.
- Up to 80 percent of patients feel relief within a week.

Disadvantages of wide-field radiation:

- It causes nausea and vomiting in 80 percent of those treated.
- It causes blood disorders in about 10 percent of patients.
- Between 10 percent and 35 percent of patients will experience inflammation of the lungs, a condition called radiation pneumonitis.

Combined drug therapy — A new pain medication for those with metastatic hormone-insensitive prostate cancer (also called hormone-refractory prostate cancer) was recently FDA approved. The drug, called Novantrone (mitoxantrone), made by Immunex Corp. of Seattle, is delivered intravenously once every three weeks in combination with prednisone, which is taken orally twice a day. The combination of these two drugs has been shown to significantly reduce cancer pain in almost a third (33 percent) of those who've taken it, as compared with patients taking prednisone alone. While Novantrone reduces cancer pain, it is not taken to extend the length of life.

FAST FACT

When deciding on the right treatment, almost half of all prostate-cancer patients are most concerned with maintaining quality of life, while three out of 10 patients (30 percent) are most concerned with having their lives extended.

The ABCs of CHAPTER 8

A Quick Review

A

What is single-agent androgen-deprivation (hormonal) therapy?

- There are two types of prostate-cancer cells: "hormone-sensitive" and "hormone-insensitive." The more hormone-sensitive cells you have, the better you'll respond to hormone therapy. The more hormone-insensitive cells you have, the less successful your results will be from such treatment.

- There are three equally effective ways to decrease testosterone levels and thus increase the quality and quantity of life: bilateral orchiectomy (surgical removal of the testicles), LHRH agonists and DES (hormonal therapy). All three treatments decrease a man's testosterone level to near zero, which cuts off the cancer's "fuel supply."

- The disadvantages of androgen-deprivation therapy include decreased sex drive, impotence, hot flashes, breast enlargement, nipple tenderness and weight gain around the midsection.

B

What is combination androgen-deprivation (complete hormonal) therapy?

- Combination therapy is when an antiandrogen drug (such as flutamide, bicalutamide or nilutamide) is used in tandem with bilateral orchiectomy (surgical removal of the testicles) or an LHRH agonist.

- For those whose prostate cancer is extremely advanced, combination androgen-deprivation therapy is of little benefit compared to single-agent androgen-deprivation therapy. However, it can prolong life by several months in men with early advanced prostate cancer whose cancer has escaped the prostate but has not yet spread throughout the body.

- Antiandrogens may need to be discontinued in some cases because of a condition called androgen-withdrawal syndrome, which can stimulate cancer growth rather than inhibit it.

- Suramin or its derivatives can be used to combat hormone-insensitive cancer cells. Suramin has shown some promise in helping a small number of individuals, but its benefits are temporary. The drug's side effects include a weakened immune system, decreased production of blood platelets (and thus clotting), pain and fatigue.

- Chemotherapy for prostate cancer has not been shown to extend the quality or quantity of life. However, combinations of chemotherapeutic drugs are being tested that show promise.

C

What are the best strategies for dealing with cancer pain?

- There is no need for any prostate cancer patient to suffer a great deal of pain. Many pain medications can be given for general pain (from aspirin to codeine to morphine). The key is to work with your doctor in effectively combating your specific type of pain.

- The best treatment for spot pain is a combination of strontium 89, an injectable drug that relieves bone pain, and spot radiation targeted to the specific pain site.

- There is no evidence to show that pain medications are addictive; in fact research has shown that pain management can increase the quality as well as the quantity of a patient's life.

Medical References

Title: **"Maximal androgen blockade for patients with metastatic prostate cancer: outcome of a controlled trial of bicalutamide versus flutamide, each in combination with luteinizing hormone-releasing hormone analogue therapy"**
Authors: Schellhammer, P.; Sharifi, R.; Block, N.; et al
Journal: *Urology*
Volume: 47 (1A Suppl)
Pages: 54-60, 80-84 (discussion)
Date: January 1996

Title: **"Megestrol acetate for the prevention of hot flashes"**
Authors: Loprinzi, C.L.; Michalak, J.C.; Quella, S.K.; et al
Journal: *New England Journal of Medicine*
Volume: 331
Pages: 347-352
Date: Aug. 11, 1994

Title: **"Pain management in the patient with prostate cancer"**
Author: Payne, R.
Journal: Cancer
Volume: 71 (3 Suppl)
Pages: 1131-1137
Date: Feb. 1, 1993

Title: **"Goserelin acetate and flutamide versus bilateral orchiectomy: a phase III EORTC trial (30853). EORTC GU and EORTC Data Center."**
Authors: Denis, L.J.; Carnelo de Moura, J.L.; Bono, A.; et al
Journal: *Urology*
Volume: 42 (2)
Pages: 119-129, 129-130 (discussion)
Date: August 1993

Title: **"A controlled trial of leuprolide with and without flutamide in protastatic carcinoma"**
Authors: Crawford, E.D.; Eisenberger, M.A.; McLeod, D.G.; et al
Journal: *New England Journal of Medicine*
Volume: 321 (7)
Pages: 419-424
Date: Aug. 17, 1989

9

Coping with the Major
Treatment Complications

A

What can I do about
urine leakage?

B

How will my sex life
be affected?

C

What can I do about bowel
(and other) complications?

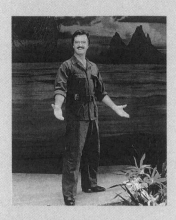

Robert Goulet
Actor

Three weeks from the day of my prostate-cancer surgery I was back in tights onstage in L.A., in a touring production of "Camelot." Worried about incontinence, I wore three pairs of shorts (with half a "Depend" wedged in there) and went out in front of all those people, singing away as though nothing was wrong.

Standing on a high mound (where most of the audience could see up my bodice), as I sang a high note in the title song, I felt a "splurt" issue from my body. Still singing, I asked myself, "Was it a big splurt or a little one? Did the audience see it or not?" I knew it was a fait accompli, so I told myself to smile and get on with the scene.

When we left the stage at the end of the scene, I turned to my leading lady, Patricia Kies, and asked her, "When I sang that high note, did you see the twinkle in my eye?" "Yes," she responded, "and when I saw that twinkle in your eye, I knew there was a tinkle down your thigh!"

Anyway, thanks to the PSA test, I'm alive and well and now I tell every 40-year-old man I know to get one. It may save a few lives!

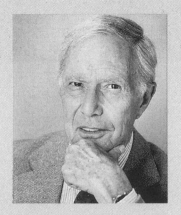

Mason Adams
Actor

One of the consequences of prostatectomy and radiation is incontinence, and for a while I had it in good measure. At the time that I was being radiated I was also doing a play in New York. The play was staged in a hospital room, and it opened with me in a pair of white pajamas doing tai chi. Here I was, suffering from incontinence, going onstage every night in white pajamas and scared out of my wits that I'd have an accident. I never did, but the circumstance was surely ironic.

As to whether there's been anything positive about my experience with prostate cancer, other than the fact that I came through it, I really can't say. But I do know a number of men who weren't as lucky as me — men who waited too long to go to the doctor and died, or whose quality of life has been severely altered by the disease. I was fortunate because my cancer was caught in time. Even after surgery and radiation therapy, the quality of my life hasn't changed too much. So I am constantly advising younger friends to be sure to go to the doctor and get examined at least once a year.

A
What can I do about urine leakage?

Bed wetting. Leakage. Dribbling. There are many names for incontinence, or loss of urinary control, probably because it is such a common problem in men and women. Incontinence affects more than 10 million Americans, but less than 10 percent of those who suffer from it seek medical attention. However, it is estimated that Americans spend $15 billion a year in the quest to stay dry.

Incontinence can occur for a number of reasons, including age and physical stress, such as lifting. Treatment for prostate cancer (radical prostatectomy and radiation therapy) also can lead to incontinence. Among men who undergo surgery for prostate cancer, in most cases the condition is temporary and resolves itself over time or can be corrected with minor treatment. However, less than 5 percent of prostatectomy patients experience severe incontinence that can only be corrected with surgery.

Regardless of the severity, the problem is usually treatable. However, it must first be diagnosed with one or more of the following five tests:

Cystogram — A test in which a tube (called a catheter) is placed through the penis into the bladder. Through this tube, the bladder is slowly filled with a type of dye that allows the doctor to view the organ upon X-ray.

Cystometrogram — A test in which a catheter is used to measure and record the bladder's average pressure as it fills with and releases urine.

Cystoscopy — A procedure in which a lighted tube (called a cystoscope) is placed inside the penis and up into the bladder so the doctor can see how well the continence-controlling muscles work.

Urinary flow rate — A test that measures the speed with which the urine leaves the penis (in milliliters per second, or ml/sec).

Urine culture — This is when a urine sample is analyzed for any bacteria that could be causing an infection, a possible explanation for urinary trouble.

There are basically five types of incontinence, all of which can be caused by prostate-cancer treatment. These types of incontinence can occur separately or together:

Overflow incontinence (also called false incontinence) — This is when the bladder never drains completely because the urethra and/or bladder neck is scarred and narrowed, or the bladder no longer contracts due to certain medications or injury. Therefore, the bladder is constantly filling with urine and the pressure becomes too great, which causes leakage. Typical symptoms of overflow incontinence include:

• being unable to urinate even though you feel the urge to go;

• getting up repeatedly at night to urinate;

• leaking small amounts of urine throughout the day;

• taking a long time to urinate and when it finally happens, the stream may be very weak; and

• feeling like your bladder is still full even after you have finished urinating.

Stress incontinence (also called anatomic incontinence) — This is when any movement or action that could put pressure on the bladder results in urine leakage. Symptoms include:

• leaking urine when you cough, laugh, sneeze or exercise;

• leaking urine upon standing from a seated position or getting out of bed; and

• needing to urinate more often so the bladder is never too full.

Urge incontinence — This is when the urge to go to the bathroom is so great, you cannot "hold it." That's because the bladder is pushing urine out with so much force that its sphincter cannot hold it back. Symptoms include:

• getting up many times at night to urinate;

• needing to urinate every few hours throughout the day; and

- wetting the bed at night or wetting yourself on the way to the bathroom.

Total incontinence — This is when the bladder constantly leaks urine, regardless of what time of day or night it is or what type of activity you're undertaking.

Mixed incontinence — This is when two or more types of incontinence occur together, such as stress and urge incontinence.

Absorbent male undergarments, or "adult diapers" as they have been called, are effective in managing leakage and are usually used as the first line of defense for those who leak in the initial months after surgery or radiation therapy. They are relatively inexpensive, save a lot of potential embarrassment and expense from soiled clothing and furniture, and most are not noticeable under clothes. There are basically four types of disposable or reusable products that absorb urine effectively:

Adult undergarments — These are the bulkiest of the protective undergarments, and they look like heavily padded underwear. They are usually worn only at night or while at home.

Adult briefs — These are less bulky than undergarments and can be worn like underwear under loose clothing.

Adult pads — These are pads that come in all degrees of thickness and they are placed inside your regular underwear. They can be worn without notice under regular clothing.

Bed or mattress pads — These cover and protect your bed or mattress while you sleep.

To prevent or lessen the severity of incontinence, some physicians have their patients do what is called the Kegel exercise (also called the special perineal exercise) before and after prostate surgery. The Kegel exercise involves strengthening the pelvic muscles by deliberately starting and stopping the urine flow. When not urinating, the same results can be achieved by tightening the muscles of the pelvis or buttocks. Regular practice of the Kegel exercise may reduce leakage or correct it permanently. This exercise should be repeated three times a day for several weeks or months. Results vary from individual to individual; some think they can cure incontinence with these exercises while others think they are useless.

There are two sets of muscles, or sphincters, that prevent urinary leakage: those at the base of the bladder (also called bladder-neck muscles or the internal sphincter) and those directly below the bladder (also called the external sphincter) that surround the urethra (the tube that carries urine from the body). If anything happens to these muscles or the nerves that control them, incontinence can result.

Radiation therapy causes long-term (greater than one year after treatment) urinary incontinence in less than 5 percent of those treated. This type of incontinence usually occurs after the radiation treatment has been completed. If the radiation damages the sphincter muscles that prevent urine leakage, the result is stress incontinence. If the radiation affects the bladder as a whole, the resulting irritation can cause urge incontinence. If both structures are affected by radiation, then both types of incontinence are likely to occur (mixed incontinence).

Radical prostatectomy, as mentioned previously, causes long-term (greater than one year after treatment) urinary incontinence in 3 percent to greater than 50 percent of those who undergo the procedure. The reason for this wide variation is because the doctor performing the surgery has a lot to do with the incontinence risk. Of course, this is not to say that whether you have incontinence after the surgery is 100-percent dependent on the surgeon. Incontinence will result in a small percentage of patients regardless of the surgeon's skill. However, it is very important to choose an experienced surgeon — one who has not only performed this surgery many times but who continues to perform it regularly (at least four times a month, in our opinion).

Cryosurgery, in which the prostate gland is frozen, also can cause freezing of the urinary sphincter, resulting in long-term incontinence in 5 percent to 15 percent of patients.

Now lets talk about the information that probably interested you in reading this chapter in the first place: how incontinence is treated. The options are both nonsurgical and surgical.

Nonsurgical treatment of incontinence

If your bladder cannot store urine properly there are a number of medications and nonsurgical procedures that may help:

Ditropan (oxybutinin) — This is one of the most popular incontinence medications (called an anticholinergic drug). The dosage is 2.5 or 5 mg two to four times a day, depending on how well the medication is tolerated. The potential side effects are usually dry mouth, feeling tired and sleepy, and heart palpitations. It should not be given to people with increased eye (intraocular) pressure (also called glaucoma).

Pro-Banthine (propantheline bromide) — This drug is usually not as effective as Ditropan but can be used along with it, and a minority of patients find it easier to tolerate. The regular dosage is 15 mg two to three times a day, and some patients take a larger dose at bedtime to prevent leakage while they sleep. The potential side effects include dry mouth, visual problems and glaucoma.

Tofranil (imipramine hydrochloride) — This drug is very effective in controlling leakage. The dosage is 10 or 25 mg two to four times daily. The potential side effects are dry mouth, constipation, blurred vision and feeling tired or sleepy.

Chlorpheniramine maleate — A widely used antihistamine, this is available in long-working 8-mg capsules or can be taken in 4-mg doses twice a day. It also can be taken with another medication called Ornade Spansules. Side effects are dry nasal passages and a dry mouth.

Muscle relaxants — Drugs such as flavoxate hydrochloride (Urispas) can be taken orally (200 mg) three to four times a day.

Catheterization (also called self-catheterization) — Some men whose bladders cannot generate a forceful contraction to urinate can be treated by regular or occasional self-catheterization. When performing self-catheterization a small, narrow tube called a catheter is placed inside the penis every four to six hours to drain the bladder of urine. This always sounds more difficult than it is, but after a few times most patients are very comfortable using a catheter. All that's required is a restroom with privacy. Men who carry their catheters with them can enjoy a wide range of normal activities.

Condom catheters and penile clamps —The condom catheter is a condom that is placed over the penis which drains any leaked urine into a bag. A penile clamp is a device that literally clamps the penis, closing the urethra from the outside to prevent urine leakage. Neither device should be used as a first-line treatment. The condom catheter can cause numerous infections, while the penile clamp can scar or damage the penis.

Surgical treatment of incontinence

Surgical treatment of incontinence should only be considered for those patients whose leakage is extreme, lasting at least a year without signs of improvement. Surgical options include:

Collagen injection — Collagen is a protein found throughout the human body. Many people have already received collagen injections to fill in scars or wrinkles. The collagen used in this procedure is derived from cows.

This minimally invasive outpatient treatment can be performed under local anesthesia. During the procedure, a cystoscope is placed into the penis and up into the bladder through which collagen is injected into the bladder neck (see Fig. 9A-1). The addition of collagen closes the opening of the bladder into the urethra, but this opening expands normally upon voluntary urination.

Three to four treatments are usually required before a successful result may be achieved. Because each injection costs several hundred dollars, when all is said and done, it is not unusual for this treatment to cost several thousand dollars.

It is important to wait at least a year after prostate surgery before considering collagen injection to make sure that the incontinence has had an ample chance to improve on its own. It is also important

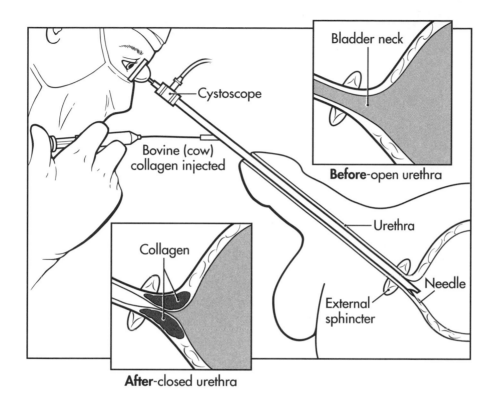

Before-open urethra

Bladder neck

Cystoscope

Bovine (cow) collagen injected

Collagen

After-closed urethra

Urethra

Needle

External sphincter

Fig. 9A-1 — Transurethral Collagen Injection

During the collagen-injection procedure, a cystoscope is placed into the penis and up into the bladder, through which collagen is injected into the bladder neck. The addition of collagen closes the opening of the bladder into the ure-thra, which prevents urine leakage. However, the urethra expands normally upon voluntary urination.

to have a skin test about a month before the surgery to rule out the chance of allergic reaction to the collagen. During a skin test, a small amount of collagen is injected into the skin of the arm to see if any redness, swelling, or itching occurs that would indicate a pos-sible sensitivity. This usually occurs in the first three days, but it can happen for up to a month. Such an allergy is extremely rare, affecting less than 1 percent of patients.

Men who experience incontinence from radiation treatment are not good candidates for collagen injections, as scar tissue caused by the radiation prevents the material from being injected properly.

Among men whose leakage is caused by surgery, collagen treatment works well in about a third of those who request it. It may work well for several months or many years — the results vary from person to person (see Table 9A-1).

Table 9A-1 — **Report Card:** *Collagen Injection*

✔ **Effectiveness**

Short-term (up to a year after treatment)

Chance of achieving total dryness	35%
Chance of partial continence improvement	40-50%

Long-term (two years after treatment)

Chance of achieving total dryness	25%
Chance of partial continence improvement	30-40%

✔ **Side effects**

Risk of temporary urinary retention immediately after treatment	8%
Risk of incontinence worsening after treatment	10%
Risk of bladder infection	4%
Risk of blood in urine	2%

✔ **Total average cost**
(Depending on number of injections needed) $2,000–10,000

The best candidates for collagen implants are:

- men with minimal incontinence (who use one to two pads daily) who have not shown improvement in their symptoms for at least a year after treatment; and
- men whose incontinence has been caused by surgery.

Advantages of collagen injection:

- The procedure is done on an outpatient basis.
- The collagen works naturally and there is nothing the patient has to do.

Disadvantages of collagen injection:

- It is not effective in men whose incontinence has been caused by radiation therapy.
- The treatment process requires multiple injections/sessions.
- The long-term effectiveness (after two years) is not known.
- The injections are expensive, with a total cost of between $2,000 and $10,000.

The artificial sphincter — This is a surgically implanted device that can be used to correct severe, long-term incontinence lasting a year or more. It consists of a cuff placed around the urethra or bladder neck. When the cuff is inflated with saline solution (manually triggered by a pump implanted in the scrotum), it squeezes shut the urethra or bladder neck and thus prevents urine leakage (see Fig. 9A-2). When the cuff is deflated, the pressure is released and urination can occur.

While complications from this device are rare, they can include infection, continued urine leakage, bleeding and mechanical malfunction (see Table 9A-2). The artificial sphincter can be implanted successfully in 95 percent of cases.

Table 9A-2 — **Report Card:** *Artificial Sphincter*

✔ **Effectiveness**	
Successful implantation rate	90-95 %
Rate of mechanical malfunction	10-35 %
Rate of surgical complications	10-35 %
✔ **Side effects**	
Risk of sphincter erosion	5-7 %
Risk of infection	5-10 %
(More long-term complication results are needed)	
✔ **Total average cost**	$12,000–$18,000

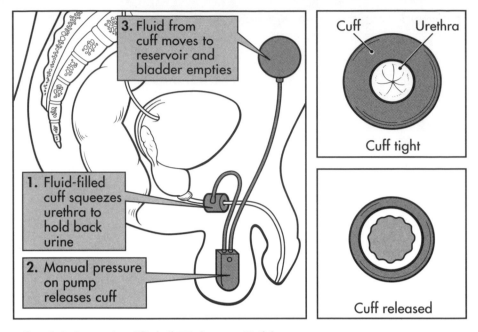

Fig. 9A-2 — Artificial Urinary Sphincter

The artificial urinary sphincter consists of a cuff that is placed around the urethra or bladder neck. When the cuff is inflated with saline (manually triggered by a pump implanted in the scrotum), it squeezes shut the urethra or bladder neck, thus blocking urine flow. When the cuff is deflated, the pressure on the urinary tract is released and urination can occur.

The operation is performed under spinal or general anesthesia and requires a one- or two-day hospital stay. Two incisions are made during surgery, the first is below the scrotum and the second in the lower abdominal area. After surgery, a catheter may be inserted to drain your bladder, but it is usually removed before you leave the hospital. A drainage tube may also be placed in the abdomen if there is excess fluid near the incision site.

The artificial sphincter itself cannot be used for the first four to six weeks after surgery, because the urethra needs this time to rest and heal. Therefore, you will remain incontinent during this period.

When you have recovered from surgery your doctor will activate the artificial sphincter, after which it can be manually controlled by you. The artificial sphincter is made from a type of rubber called silicone elastomer, which is not a silicone gel. There is no evidence in the medical literature that this type of silicone causes an allergic reaction.

The best candidates for artificial sphincters are:
- men with severe incontinence (who use three pads or more daily) whose symptoms have not improved for at least a year.

Advantages of the artificial sphincter:
- It is the most effective treatment for severe, long-term incontinence.
- It is easy to use.

Disadvantages of the artificial sphincter:
- There is a long-term risk of mechanical failure, requiring replacement.
- It requires a one- to two-day hospital stay.
- It is expensive, costing an average total of $12,000 to $18,000.

FAST FACT

Encouraging long-term research on a double-cuff urinary sphincter device has just been released, showing a greater than 95-percent success rate over a nine-year period.

B

How will my sex life be affected?

"Erectile dysfunction" is another fancy medical term but it just means that a man has trouble in the erection department. He may not be able to stay erect very long, he may not be able to achieve an erection every time, or his erections may not be as strong as they were before treatment.

Causes of erectile dysfunction

There are basically five treatments for prostate cancer, each of which can cause erectile dysfunction or impotence:

Watchful waiting — Erectile problems among men who practice watchful waiting are uncommon, but they do occur. Their cause is unclear. The tumor maybe growing and invading the nerves that control erection (these nerves are located near the prostate), or the mental stress some individuals experience after being told they have cancer may cause sexual difficulty.

Radiation therapy — In targeting cancerous tissue in or near the prostate, external-beam radiation therapy and radioactive-seed implantation can sometimes damage the nerves that help a man have an erection or control blood flow to the penis. Between 20 percent and 30 percent of men undergoing radiation therapy experience impotence. *Treatment:* See list of interventions on Page 187.

Radical prostatectomy (surgery) — There are two bundles of nerves on each side of the prostate that act like switches that activate an erection. If both are removed or damaged, then you will have erectile problems. If one or both bundles are left intact, it is possible to continue having erections as strong as they were before the surgery. However, more than half of those who undergo radical prostatectomy may experience some degree of impotence afterward. Again, look for an experienced surgeon like you would an experienced mechanic, a person who not only has experience but continues to do the procedure on a regular basis and with good results. This could definitely affect your chances of remaining potent.

There are also some factors that cannot be helped by the surgeon. Erectile function after surgery also depends on your age, the strength of your erections before surgery, and the amount of cancer and degree to which it has spread before surgery. Younger men with smaller tumors have the best chance of retaining normal erections. *Treatment:* See list below.

Androgen-deprivation therapy — Men undergoing androgen-deprivation therapy, whose testosterone levels have been greatly reduced, may lose the desire to have intercourse (decreased libido) or may not be able to have an erection. The male hormones help create the desire for sex, so although the nerves and the blood supply to the penis are all in working order, the desire to have an erection may not be there. *Treatment:* There are no interventions that can restore normal libido as long as you remain on hormonal therapy.

Cryosurgery (freezing of the prostate) — Because the nerves around the prostate are frozen during this procedure, most men (90 percent) who undergo cryosurgery cannot have an erection afterward. *Treatment:* None. However, in a small percentage of cryosurgery patients (10 percent) the nerves recover from the injury and erectile function returns.

Treatments for erectile dysfunction

There are a variety of interventions for men whose erectile dysfunction is associated with prostate-cancer treatment (see Table 9B). They include:

Medication — There is a tablet that can be taken that helps with erectile problems in a very small percentage of patients. It is called Yokon (Yohimbine HCL). One 5.4-mg tablet is taken three times a day. This drug can cause nausea, dizziness, and/or nervousness in some patients. If this occurs the dosage should be reduced or the patient should be taken off the drug.

By the end of the century a promising pill for treating impotence (made by Pfizer) should be available.

Penile self-injections — This involves using a tiny needle and syringe to inject medication into the side of the penis (see Fig. 9B-1). The drug causes blood to flow into the areas of the penis called the corpus cavernosa and the corpus spongiosum, which produces a strong erection. While the idea of putting a needle into the penis may sound about as attractive as having multiple root canals on the same day, patients are usually surprised at how simple and painless this procedure can be.

The medications used include one or more of the following: phentolamine, papaverine or PGE (prostaglandin E). Patients have little difficulty learning from their doctor how to draw the right amount of medication and inject it properly. It takes only about 10 minutes

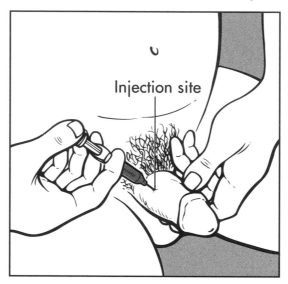

Fig. 9B-1 — Pharmacologic Therapy (Penile Self-injection)

In penile self-injection, the patient injects a drug into the side of his penis, which causes blood to flow into the organ, producing a strong erection.

for the medication to work, and the resulting erection usually lasts at least 30 minutes. The cost is about $100 for as many as 15 to 20 injections, and most insurance companies will cover the expense.

The prospect of a 30-minute erection may sound fantastic, but there's a catch: Injections must be limited to three times a week to prevent the risk of injuring or scarring the penis. Also, in a small number of cases, injections can cause a condition called priapism, in which the erection continues for a long but unhealthy period of time. Because the blood in the penis is trapped, it thickens due to loss of oxygen, which can damage the penile tissue. If priapism occurs, placing a towel-covered ice pack over the penis usually solves the problem. If, despite the ice pack, the erection doesn't go away, a doctor should be called immediately because this is considered an emergency.

The proper dosage for injection is determined by trial and error. Some patients require a small dosage while others require a large amount of the drug to develop and maintain an erection. It is essential for the patient and the doctor to determine the proper dosage before self-injection can begin. If the man's partner wants to give the injection this is also encouraged, because it can actually be stimulating for both parties to incorporate this into foreplay.

A gel that can be rubbed on the penis for the treatment of impotence may soon gain FDA approval. This gel, made by MacroChem, contains the same active ingredient used in penile injection therapy.

Testosterone injections — While these have received some attention, they should not be given to treat erectile problems after prostate surgery because testosterone could encourage the growth of any prostate-cancer cells that could be left in the body. STAY AWAY FROM THESE TYPES OF INJECTIONS.

Vacuum constriction devices — These apparatuses consist of a large plastic tube, a pump, lubrication and a rubber band or elastic ring. The tube is placed over the lubricated penis and the pump is used to create a vacuum, or suction, inside the tube, which causes blood to flow into the penis and a strong erection to result. The ring or rubber band is then taken off the tube and placed around the bottom of the penis to keep the blood inside the organ so that the erection can be maintained (see Fig. 9B-2). The erection ends when the band or ring is removed (up to 30 minutes later) by the man or his partner. The great thing about this device is that it can work in patients who have nerve damage because it manually brings blood into the penis. And, as long as this device is not used for more than 30 minutes at a time, it can be used several times a week.

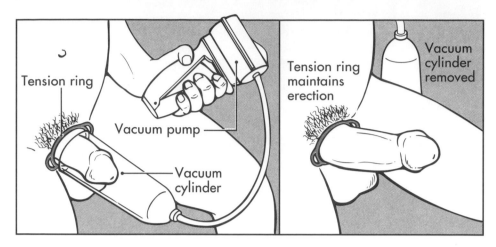

Fig. 9B-2 — Vacuum Constriction Device

This technique involves the use of vacuum, or suction, to draw blood into the penis and produce an erection. Once the penis is erect, a ring or rubber band is placed around the base of the penis to keep the blood inside the organ. The erection lasts as long as the band is in place.

Potential drawbacks of the vacuum device: Some patients feel that the ring or elastic band is uncomfortable and the penis feels colder because there is no blood circulation. Others complain that it looks unnatural to wear the ring or use the device. Regardless, it is effective and the companies that make it usually have videos and sales representatives who can answer any questions and handle any concerns. A good device can cost up to $500, but Medicare and many insurance companies will cover some of the cost. Most also come with a trial period and a money-back guarantee. A doctor's prescription is needed for this device.

Penile implants (prostheses) — These are another popular solution for erectile problems. While implants don't allow the head of the penis to swell as well as it would naturally, they are still effective in producing an erection.

There are four types of penile prostheses:

- **The malleable, or bendable, implant** — also called the semi-rigid penile prosthesis (see Fig. 9B-3) — this is the easiest to implant and the least likely to malfunction. It is a collection of wires within a silicone covering. Once implanted, the penis stays erect constantly with this device, which is manually adjusted.

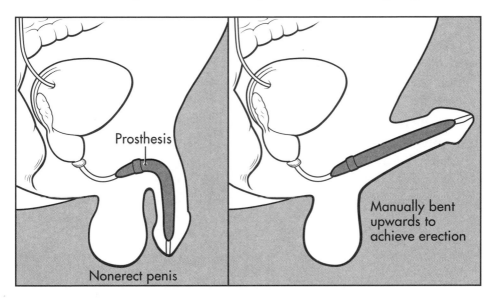

Prosthesis

Nonerect penis

Manually bent upwards to achieve erection

Fig. 9B-3 — Malleable Penile Implant

This penile implant consists of a collection of wires within a silicone covering. Once surgically implanted, the penis stays erect constantly and can be manually adjusted upward or downward.

- **The mechanical implant** — a spring-loaded steel cable encased in a series of interlocking plastic blocks, this is very similar to the malleable implant above, except the penis does not become erect until the device is manually locked in place. In addition, it is easier to bend — a plus for people who are not as strong with their hands, such as those with arthritis.

- **Inflatable implant without pump** — when the tip of this device is squeezed in the glans (head) of the penis it causes fluid within the implant to shift around and the penis then becomes hard. When the implant is bent and a release valve is used, the erection subsides.

- **Inflatable implant with pump** — this provides the most natural erection of any of the devices (see Fig. 9B-4). In addition to an implant, a pump is placed into the scrotum between the testicles. When the pump is squeezed, it allows fluid to flow into the implant, thus causing an erection. Since this is a more complicated device, there is the slight chance of complication that may require additional surgery to repair.

All of the above implants are inserted into the penis through either an incision directly into the penis or in the lower abdominal wall. Most of these procedures can be done on an outpatient basis. One must wait about four to six weeks after the surgery before resuming intercourse. This time is needed for the area to heal. Implants are meant to be permanent; if removed, erection will be impossible by any other means.

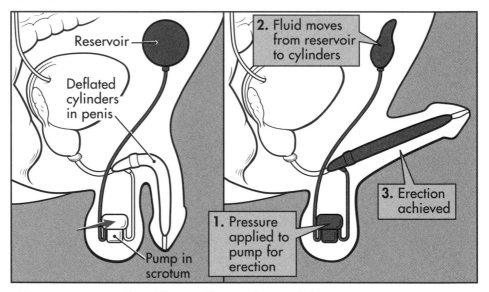

Fig. 9B-4 — Inflatable Penile Implant with Pump

This provides the most natural erection of any of the devices, allowing the penis to be flaccid (limp) as well as erect. When an erection is desired, a pump implanted into the scrotum is squeezed; this sends fluid into the implant, which produces an erection.

Complications of implants can include infection, which requires antibiotic therapy and/or removal of the device; erosion, in which the implant can extend through the urethra or even the side of the penis; torque, in which the wires of the implant can twist on each other causing the penis to twist; pain, which can be treated with medication; and general malfunction or the need for replacement.

Depending on the implant chosen, the price can range from a few thousand dollars to $20,000 for the device and the operation to implant it. The more technical the implant, the greater the price. Many insurance companies cover the cost of these devices.

Table 9B — Surgical and Nonsurgical Treatments
for Impotence: the Pros and Cons

COUNSELING/SEX THERAPY

Advantages

No surgery or drugs. Leads to understanding of true emotional needs. Improves communication with partner.

Disadvantages

Therapy required for indeterminate time. Success rates vary. Hourly costs ranges $75-$150.

TOPICAL VASODILATORS

Advantages

Nonsurgical. Painless. Easy to apply.

Disadvantages

Condom required to protect partner from side effects. No reports on long-term use. May cause headaches. Costs about $15-$30 monthly.

ORAL MEDICATIONS

Advantages

Nonsurgical. Painless. May improve libido.

Disadvantages

Minimal effectiveness. Treatment must continue as long as sexual activity desired. Side effects include dizziness, nausea, nervousness and headaches. Cost about $15-$30 monthly.

Continued

Table 9B (cont'd) — Surgical and Nonsurgical Treatments for Impotence: the Pros and Cons

HORMONE REPLACEMENT

Advantages

Nonsurgical. Painless. May improve libido.

Disadvantages

Effective only when cause is severe testosterone deficiency. Can stimulate growth of prostatic tissue, cause liver damage or tumors, stop sperm production and increase generalized fluid retention. Costs about $25-$35 monthly.

EXTERNAL VACUUM THERAPY

Advantages

Safe. Nonsurgical. Use as often as desired. Will not interfere with other treatments. May improve penile blood flow and result in spontaneous erection. Over 90-percent success rate.

Disadvantages

Requires some manual dexterity and strength. Tension ring should be removed within 30 minutes. Involves learning a manual technique. Mild bruising may occur, usually when learning. Costs $400-$600. Annual cost of lubricant and tension ring: $30-$50.

PENILE INJECTION THERAPY

Advantages

Nonsurgical. Rapid erectile response in about 70 percent of cases. Erection lasts one to two hours. One or more drugs may be combined to reduce discomfort and risks.

Disadvantages

Requires test dosing and follow-up by urologist. Drugs used are not approved by the FDA for penile injection. Frequency of use limited to two to three times per week. Fibrosis or scaring may occur. Prolonged painful erection may require "antidote" or surgical intervention. Annual cost: $500-$1,500.

SEMI-RIGID PENILE PROSTHESES

Advantages

Simple device. Less expensive than inflatable models. Shorter surgical time. No mechanical parts to break down. High success rates.

Disadvantages

Requires a surgical procedure. Permanent erection, but concealable. Medical or device failure is possible due to infection, rejection or mechanical failure. Permanently alters internal structure of penis and may preclude other treatment. Costs more than nonsurgical treatments. Costs approximately $6,000.

Table 9B (cont'd)

SELF-CONTAINED INFLATABLE AND MECHANICAL PROSTHESES

Advantages

Controllable natural-appearing erection. Easily concealed. Very effective. Less expensive than multi-component inflatable prostheses.

Disadvantages

Requires a surgical procedure. Higher incidence of mechanical failure than semi-rigid prostheses due to infection, rejection or mechanical failure. Does not allow full girth of penis. Permanently alters internal structure of penis and may preclude other treatment. Cost approximately $6,000-$10,000.

MULTI-COMPONENT INFLATABLE PENILE PROSTHESES

Advantages

Controllable, natural-appearing erection. Full girth and true flaccidity. Easily concealed. High patient/partner satisfaction.

Disadvantages

Requires a surgical procedure. Higher cost than simple prostheses and nonsurgical treatments. Longer surgical time. Medical or device failure is possible due to infection, rejection or mechanical failure. Permanently alters internal structure of penis and may preclude other treatment. Costs approximately $6,000-$12,000.

RECONSTRUCTION VENOUS LIGATION

Advantages

Effective when the problem is due to vascular obstruction or deformity.

Disadvantages

Sophisticated surgical procedure. Effective for only about 1 percent of patients. Very high relapse rate. Very high cost, approximately $15,000.

Source: Geddings-Obson Sr. Foundation.

FAST FACT

Less than 10 percent of men who suffer from impotence seek medical attention.

C

What can I do about bowel (and other) complications?

A small number — between 10 percent and 20 percent — of patients who undergo radiation therapy experience bowel complications or problems with the stomach, intestines or rectum. It is difficult to avoid exposing the bowel or rectum to radiation at least a little, since the rectum lies right behind the prostate (see Fig. 9C). However, the chance of bowel problems can be decreased significantly if an individual is treated by an experienced radiation oncologist. Bowel problems can also result after a radical prostatectomy, but as with radiation, they affect only a small percentage of patients.

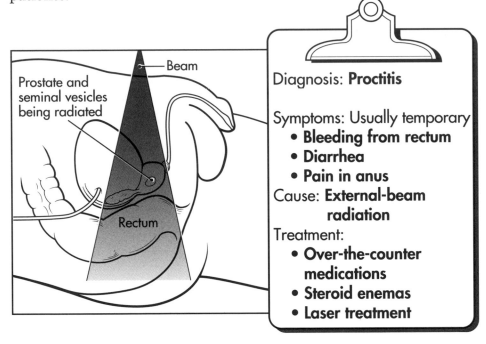

Prostate and seminal vesicles being radiated

Beam

Rectum

Diagnosis: **Proctitis**

Symptoms: Usually temporary
- **Bleeding from rectum**
- **Diarrhea**
- **Pain in anus**

Cause: **External-beam radiation**

Treatment:
- **Over-the-counter medications**
- **Steroid enemas**
- **Laser treatment**

Fig. 9C — Radiation-induced Proctitis

External-beam radiation therapy is extremely accurate today; however, it is difficult to block the bowel or rectum from radiation because it lies right behind the prostate. This exposure can result in radiation-induced proctitis, or inflammation of the rectum.

There are also certain uncontrollable factors that can increase one's chances of having bowel problems, such as tumor size. The larger the tumor, the more radiation is needed and the greater the risk of bowel problems.

Below is a list of the most common bowel problems associated with prostate-cancer treatment, as well as their potential remedies. All of these complications can occur for a few weeks to several months after treatment and most will eventually go away on their own. (For a list of other complications and their treatments, see Table 9C.)

Diarrhea — Loose bowel movements can be treated by taking an oral medication such as Imodium.

Blood in the stool — Mild cases can be treated with stool softeners, steroid enemas and anti-inflammatory drugs. If the bleeding continues, this can be due to a more serious rectal ulcer (an opening in the rectum), which can be treated with laser surgery.

Cramps or constipation — Cramps can be treated with a variety of prescription drugs or over-the-counter medications such as milk of magnesia.

Fecal urgency — The sensation of wanting to have a bowel movement when one does not actually need to. This can be treated by "bulking agents" such as Metamucil.

FAST FACT

Most bowel complications can be effectively treated with over-the-counter medications.

Table 9C — Other Possible Treatment Complications and Their Treatments

Complication	Treatment
Bladder-neck contracture	Dilation in the doctor's office
Deep-vein thrombosis (DVT)	Elevate legs Take blood thinners
Epididymitis	Support scrotum Take hot baths Take antibiotics
Hematuria	Lie down Drink extra water Call the doctor
Lymphocele	Take diuretics Insert drainage tube
Nausea/vomiting	Stop eating Lie down Take Compazine
Penile pain	Take pain medication
Pulmonary embolus	Take blood thinners
Rectal fistula	Insert drainage catheter Repair surgically
Scrotal swelling	Support scrotum
Testicular pain	Take hot baths Support scrotum
Thigh numbness	Resolves in 6-12 months
Urine leakage	Insert drainage catheter for 4-6 weeks
Urinary tract infections (UTIs)	Take antibiotics
Wound incision infection	Apply hot compress Take antibiotics

The ABCs of CHAPTER 9
A Quick Review

A

What can I do about urine leakage?

- There are three to five types of incontinence caused by prostate-cancer treatment: mixed, overflow, stress, urge and total incontinence.

- The first line of treatment for incontinence is usually nonsurgical. A variety of anticholinergic drugs can be prescribed, or regular or occasional self-catheterization can be used to control the risk of accidents.

- The second type of treatment for incontinence is surgical. An artificial sphincter can be implanted, or a series of collagen injections can be given.

B

How will my sex life be affected?

- Erectile problems can occur from any type of treatment for prostate cancer.

- Erectile function depends on two bundles of nerves near the prostate. If at least one of these two bundles can be spared, then it is possible to save at least some erectile function.

- Erectile problems can be treated by self-injections into the side of the penis with a prescribed medication, using a vacuum erection device, a penile implant, or an oral medication.

C

What can I do about bowel (and other) complications?

- The majority of bowel complications come from radiation therapy (10 percent to 20 percent of patients). Bowel complications can also occur in a small percentage of patients who have surgery.

- Most of the bowel difficulties go away after several months and/or can be effectively treated by over-the-counter medications.

- Less common complications of prostate-cancer treatment (such as urinary-tract infections, pain, nausea and vomiting) either go away on their own or can be treated by temporary lifestyle changes, over-the-counter products, medications or surgical repair.

Medical References

Title: **"Transurethral collagen injections in the therapy of post-radical prostatectomy incontinence"**
Authors: Cummings, J.M.; Boullier, J.A.; and Parra, R.O.
Journal: *Journal of Urology*
Volume: 155 (3)
Pages: 1011-1013
Date: March 1996

Title: **"The artificial urinary sphincter for post-radical prostatectomy incontinence: impact on urinary symptoms and quality of life"**
Authors: Fleshner, N.; and Herschorn, S.
Journal: *Journal of Urology*
Volume: 155 (4)
Pages: 1260-1264
Date: April 1996

Title: **"Proctitis after conventional external radiation therapy for prostate cancer: importance of minimizing posterior rectal dose"**
Authors: Cho, K.H.; Lee, C.K.; and Levitt, S.H.
Journal: *Radiology*
Volume: 195 (3)
Pages: 699-703
Date: June 1995

Title: **"Twelve-month comparison of two treatments for erectile dysfunction: self-injection versus external vacuum devices"**
Authors: Turner, L.A.; Althof, S.E.; Levine, S.B.; et al
Journal: *Urology*
Volume: 39 (2)
Pages: 139-144
Date: February 1992

Title: **"Diagnostic and therapeutic technology assessment. Penile implants for erectile impotence."**
Authors: No author listed
Journal: *Journal of the American Medical Association (JAMA)*
Volume: 260 (7)
Pages: 997-1000
Date: Aug. 18, 1988

Notes _____

_____

_____

_____

_____

_____

_____

_____

_____

_____

_____

_____

_____

_____

_____

_____

_____

_____

_____

10

Talking to Your Doctor: There's No Such Thing as a Dumb Question

A

How can I get the most
out of my doctor visit?

B

What are the most common questions
(uncommonly asked) about diagnosis and treatment?

C

What are some of the most common questions
(uncommonly asked) about experimental treatments?

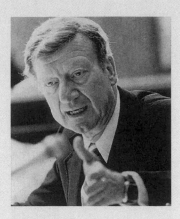

Bill Roth
U.S. senator

I can't overstate how important awareness is when it comes to cancer. Right now, education is the most, if not the only, effective way to treat prostate cancer — education that encourages early detection. We have to spread the word that, in many instances, cancer is curable, but it must be treated and detected in its early stages. My fight against prostate cancer is a success story only because I discovered it early and treated it quickly.

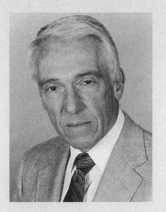

Marv Levy
Professional football coach
(Buffalo Bills)

During my annual physical, which included digital-rectal exam and a blood test for PSA screening, my doctor noticed a slightly elevate PSA score. He suggested I see a urologist, and followed his advice. The results of a sonogram administered by my urologist were negative, but a biopsy revealed that I did have prostate cancer.

I sought a second and then a third opinion ar verified that indeed I did have prostate cance. I had experienced no previous symptoms.

During the next several weeks I did a lot of research and listened carefully to valid medical advice and opinions. After considering a options I decided on surgical removal of my prostate. Three weeks after undergoing surger I was able to return to my full-time coaching duties.

My recent PSA score was 0, and I am encouraged that I am cured of this disease. The phys cal exam saved my life. I urge all men to undergo such an examination on an annual basis. It could save your life.

A

How can I get the most out of my doctor visit?

The key to a good doctor visit can be found in the word "P-R-O-S-T-A-T-E." We hope you find the following memory device helpful:

P. R. O. S. T. A. T. E.

| Preparation | Realistic expectations | Opinions | Spousal support | Take notes | Ask | Talk | Evaluate |

Preparation. Read a number of articles or books about prostate cancer before seeing your doctor. Review your medical insurance. Does it cover the cost of any experimental treatments? Does it pay for all medications and tests? If not, how much does your insurance cover? Unfortunately for most, medical costs are an important equation in the treatment decision-making process.

By doing your homework, you will develop a foundation of knowledge that will allow you to use your visit most effectively instead of having the doctor spend the valuable clinic time explaining things you could have learned on your own. Knowledge is power when it comes to prostate cancer, so the more information you have before your visit, the more you'll benefit during and after.

Realistic **Expectations.** When it comes to prostate cancer, if a treatment sounds too good to be true, then it definitely is. Always find out the disadvantages — what the "catch" is — for a specific treatment before making any decision. Insist that your doctor emphasize the cons and well as the pros of a particular treatment.

Opinions. Seek out as many opinions as possible. Do not take one person's advice as gospel, whether that person is a friend, a doctor or a member of the media. There are many different ways to play the prostate-cancer game, and to help you win, it doesn't hurt to listen to as many voices as you can before coming to your own informed decision.

Also get information from a support group or attend a meeting. Many times the meetings will have guest speakers who provide free, up-to-date medical information. Talk to the group members or at least a few patients who have gone through a similar experience. If your doctor gives you a list of patients to talk to that's fine, but also seek out patients not on that list. Even if you don't have prostate cancer, you should feel free to take advantage of such resources to learn as much as possible about the disease and its treatment.

Spousal support. Bring your spouse or partner, a family member or a friend with you to the doctor. Having someone there helps not only emotionally but mentally — by bringing up questions you may not have thought about, or by remembering something the doctor said that you could have forgotten. Also, talk to your doctor about how this process may affect your loved one and what that person can do to help make the situation better. You should also encourage your spouse or significant other to talk to others who have been in a similar situation to gain insight on how to best cope with caring for a man with prostate cancer (or in learning what a woman experiences when her husband or significant other has been diagnosed).

Take Notes. Bring a pad of paper and a pen to the doctor's office for taking notes. Bringing a tape recorder is a good idea, too.

Ask. Bring a list of questions. The ones in the next two sections of this chapter, as well as the list in Chapter 7, Section A, are a good starting point. Arriving with a list greatly increases your chances of leaving with the information you need.

Talk. Don't be afraid to tell your doctor what is on your mind. And don't be afraid to ask what you fear may be a dumb or embarrassing question. When it comes to your health, there is no such thing. You may feel uncomfortable asking questions about matters such as sexual functioning and incontinence, but such topics are routine for your doctor.

Evaluate. After collecting information from your doctor, family, friends, medical journals and books, you will end up with many, many pieces of the prostate-cancer puzzle. Sit down with your spouse, partner or a trusted friend and take time to evaluate what you have gathered. Gradually put the pieces together until the puzzle is complete. If there are still some pieces missing — if you're not sure about the effectiveness of a certain treatment or something is still unclear, go get the answer. Don't make any decisions until the puzzle is 100-percent complete.

B

What are the most common questions (uncommonly asked) about diagnosis and treatment?

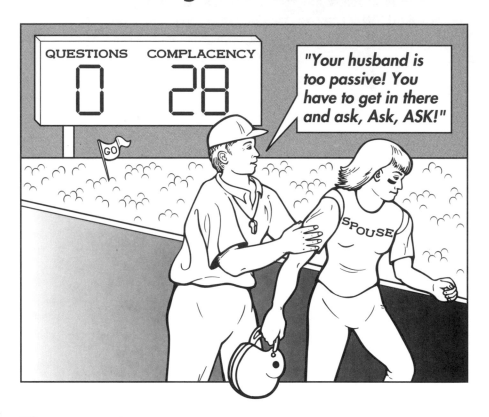

The prostate exam

1)   I don't have a family history of prostate cancer, but I do have relatives who have had other types of cancer (breast, lung, etc.) Does this mean I should start getting my prostate examined by age 40?

No. Current research points to a weak or nonexistent link between other types of cancer in the family and prostate-cancer risk. Therefore, you can wait until age 50 — unless, of course, you are black.

2) **No one in my family has died of prostate cancer, although a few had been diagnosed before death. Does this mean I should start my annual prostate checkups at age 40?**

If you are expected to live at least 10 more years, the answer is yes. A family history of prostate cancer includes being diagnosed with the disease or being suspected of having it — not just dying from it.

3) **I am not sure what some of my family members died of exactly, so I don't know whether there's a history of prostate cancer in my family. At what age should I begin having annual prostate checkups?**

If you are not sure, then you should begin at age 40, just to be on the safe side.

4) **I am black, with no family history of cancer, prostate or otherwise. Should I still get my first prostate checkup at 40?**

Absolutely. You may have no family history, but racially you are still in the highest risk group so you need to go in at 40.

6) **Can I have intercourse or ejaculate the night before my prostate exam?**

We suggest that you do not have intercourse or ejaculate for two days (48 hours) before your prostate exam to make sure that your results will be as accurate as possible.

7) **Do I have to stop drinking, smoking or eating fatty foods before my prostate exam?**

No lifestyle changes are necessary before the exam except for abstaining from ejaculation for 48 hours. Of course, it would be smart to reduce or eliminate any of the above habits to keep you in the best possible health.

8) **Is it OK to get a prostate exam while experiencing bowel problems such as diarrhea or constipation?**
Yes.

9) **Can I get a free prostate exam?**

Possibly. Check with local hospitals, especially during Prostate Cancer Awareness Week (usually the third week in September), the week of Father's Day, or check with your local public health facility.

10) **Can prostate exams be purchased as a gift for a loved one (as a gift certificate)?**

Yes. Most doctors are happy to arrange such a gift. It is an unusual idea, but a very good one.

11) **Do I have to wear a hospital gown during my prostate exam?**

No. You can wear your regular clothes; you'll just be asked to lower your pants for a few moments.

12) **If my doctor does not give me a PSA test, can I request one? How about an ultrasound?**

When it comes to the PSA test, you absolutely have the right to request one. If your doctor refuses, then find another doctor. The ultrasound, however, has not been shown to be of any great benefit if you are already having both a rectal exam and PSA test. An ultrasound is typically used only if cancer is suspected.

13) **I have heard that the PSA test can have an error margin of up to 10 percent. Should I ask for more than one PSA test?**

One PSA test per year is sufficient unless the doctor suspects a problem. In this case, the test can be repeated semi-annually.

14) **Can I get a copy of the results of my annual prostate exam?**

Absolutely. We encourage it so that you know your situation as well as anyone, and in case you change doctors or live somewhere else part of the year, you can more easily share the information with your other doctor(s).

15) **Are any institutions yet offering the new PSA "molecular forms" test (percent-free PSA test)?**

Yes, but you have to request it and there may be an additional charge.

The transrectal ultrasound (TRUS)-guided biopsy

16) **Do I have to be on antibiotics or have an enema before or after the biopsy?**

Yes. Generally, you start taking antibiotics the evening before the procedure, and the antibiotics are continued for two to three days afterwards. An enema is usually taken just prior to the biopsy to empty the rectum.

17) **What are the side effects of a biopsy?**

A transrectal ultrasound-guided biopsy of the prostate is a simple procedure that takes approximately five to 10 minutes. There is little discomfort, and the side effects are minimal. The most common side effects are developing an infection or having some bleeding from a small blood vessel that might be nicked during the biopsy procedure. Thus, it is important to take antibiotics before and after the biopsy to prevent infection, and to stop taking all medications that can thin your blood, such as aspirin, Coumadin, and any anti-inflammatory agent such as Motrin (ibuprofen).

18) **Can some prostate cancer cells become "loose" from the biopsy and go into my bloodstream and possibly grow somewhere else?**

No. The cells that are not removed stay intact within the prostate.

19) **Can I have intercourse or ejaculate right before or after the biopsy?**

There are no restrictions with regard to having sexual intercourse prior to a prostate biopsy. However, it is a good idea to abstain from ejaculation for two to three days afterward. It should also be noted that for a month to six weeks after a prostate biopsy there may be blood in the ejaculate.

20) **Can I have unprotected sex after a biopsy? Is my partner in danger of receiving some of my cancerous cells, and can they grow inside my partner's body?**

Yes, you can have unprotected sex after a biopsy. No cancer cells will escape from your body; even if they did, they could not grow inside your partner.

21) **How many samples of tissue should be taken in a biopsy?**

Most urologists will take six cores of tissue when performing a prostate biopsy. However, some will take fewer and some will take more, up to eight. The number of cores that are collected depends upon the urologist's individual practice pattern, the size of the prostate gland and the degree of PSA elevation.

22) **Besides a biopsy, is there any other way to officially confirm whether I have prostate cancer?**

No. Right now a biopsy is the only definite way.

23) **The biopsy showed high-grade PIN. Does this mean I have to have another biopsy?**

Yes. You must have repeat biopsies until the presence of cancer is either confirmed or ruled out. If repeat biopsies reveal low-grade PIN or no cancer at all, you need to return for your next prostate checkup in six months to a year. If repeat biopsies confirm the presence of cancer, treatment options are then considered.

After diagnosis

24) **Can my Gleason score be wrong, or is it 100-percent accurate?**

Your Gleason score is an opinion based on the pathologist's experience. It can vary a little according to who reads your slides. If you are not comfortable with one pathologist's opinion, you should have another pathologist confirm your Gleason score.

25) **Is it better to know my cancer's clinical stage or pathological stage?**

It is better to know your pathological stage, but this can only be determined after surgery, when your prostate tissue can be examined directly. Otherwise, the clinical stage, which is a prediction, can be accurate if the doctor uses your DRE findings, PSA level, Gleason score and other tests to determine your cancer's aggressiveness.

26) **Can I have unprotected sex after being diagnosed with prostate cancer? Is my partner in danger of receiving some of my cancerous cells, and can they grow inside my partner's body?**

Again, there is no danger of giving your partner cancer through sex or any other method.

Watchful waiting

27) **How often do I need to return to the doctor to have a rectal exam and a PSA test?**

After being diagnosed with prostate cancer and deciding to proceed with watchful waiting, it is reasonable to undergo a prostate checkup every three months for the first year. If there are no significant changes in either the PSA blood level or the DRE findings, the interval can then be lengthened to every six months.

28) **Now that I've been diagnosed with prostate cancer, will I ever need to have another prostate biopsy?**

Not usually. However, some physicians perform regular biopsies during watchful waiting to get a good idea of how your cancer is acting and whether you should start receiving treatment.

29) **Can I travel during this period and also be under the care of other doctors?**

Yes.

30) **If I decide on watchful waiting, is it true I can still undergo any traditional or experimental treatment at a later date?**

Depending on your age and overall health, your treatment options are practically unlimited as long as the cancer is confined to the prostate. Once it becomes locally advanced, however, you are no longer a candidate for radical prostatectomy.

External-beam radiation treatment

31) **Do I have to change my diet, have an enema, or take any antibiotics before or after each radiation treatment?**

No. There are few to no lifestyle changes you need to make before, during or after radiation treatment. However, it is not uncommon to alter your diet somewhat during and after radiation therapy. You may be asked to limit high-fiber foods that could irritate the rectum — such as salad, seeds, corn and apples — during and after treatment.

32) **Will I receive any type of anesthesia before this procedure?**

No. This is not an invasive procedure and it is completely painless. All you do is lie still for 15 to 30 minutes.

33) **Since I am getting radiation, is it safe for my family and friends to come near me after each daily procedure?**

Yes.

34) **Can I have intercourse or ejaculate before or after each daily procedure?**

Yes.

35) **Can I drive myself to and from the hospital after each treatment session?**

Yes.

36) **Can I leave my jewelry, rings and watch on during the treatment?**

Yes. However, it is a good idea to keep these objects out of the radiation beam.

37) **Can I read, write or listen to music during the treatment?**

It is possible to read or listen to music during the procedure. However, since you are lying on your back during treatment, it is not possible to write. Also, each session only lasts 15-30 minutes on average; therefore, you may not have enough time to read.

38) **Can I leave all of my clothes on during treatment?**

No. You will usually be asked to remove all your clothes from the waist down. However, you will be covered during the procedure by a gown or sheet.

39) **Can I work or exercise before or after each daily treatment?**

Yes. You can maintain your normal activities while undergoing daily treatment as long as your energy level allows.

40) **Can I take a little vacation during the procedure and finish the rest of my sessions when I come back?**

Yes. Radiation oncologists frequently will give a patient three weeks of radiation therapy(except weekends), a week off, and conclude with three more weeks of treatment (except weekends). This gives your pelvic organs a "breather" from the radiation. Some physicians feel that this helps reduce side effects. However, other radiation oncologists will have a patient go through six straight weeks of radiation without a break (except weekends).

41) If the first round of external-beam radiation therapy is not effective, can I go through another series of radiation treatments? Can I have radioactive seeds implanted in my prostate? Am I still eligible for surgery, cryosurgery or other treatments?

After undergoing external-beam radiation therapy (six to seven weeks of treatment), it is not possible to receive another course of external-beam therapy. It is possible, however, to undergo radical prostatectomy, cryosurgery, radioactive-seed implantation or hormonal therapy after receiving external-beam radiation therapy.

Radical prostatectomy

42) Do I have to change my diet, have an enema or take any antibiotics before or after the surgery?

No. However, after surgery you should take precautions so that your bowel movements remain soft and easy. Remember, during radical prostatectomy, the prostate gland is "peeled away" from the rectum, which is located directly behind the gland. Because the rectal wall may be traumatized slightly during the procedure, you should avoid straining during bowel movements after surgery.

43) Is there anything I can do before or after the surgery to increase my chances of a better outcome or faster recovery?

Yes. It is wise to take one to two iron pills (324 mg of ferrous sulfate or ferrous glutamate) each day from the time you decide upon surgery until you have the operation. Also during this time, it is wise to perform Kegel exercises to increase the strength of the external urinary sphincter. This is done by stopping the urinary stream in the middle of urination two to three times a day.

44) Can I have intercourse or ejaculate before or after the surgery?

While you can have sexual intercourse up until surgery, you must wait until you have recovered sufficiently before resuming sexual activities. After such surgery, it may take as long as a year for normal erections to return.

45) **Do I have to stop drinking, smoking or eating fatty foods before or after surgery?**

No. However, it is always wise to avoid these habits to maintain the best possible health.

46) **Since there are two types of radical prostatectomy (retropubic and perineal), is one better than the other?**

There are advantages and disadvantages to both techniques. With the retropubic approach, an incision is made in the lower abdomen from the navel down to the pubic bone. This allows the urologic oncologist to remove the pelvic lymph nodes and confirm that there has been no spread of the cancer. It is our opinion that one can more effectively save the nerves that control erection with this approach. Thus, the potency rate after a radical retropubic prostatectomy may be slightly better than after a radical perineal prostatectomy. The advantages of the radical perineal prostatectomy is that there is no incision in the lower abdomen, less bleeding, and heavier men fare better with this approach. As a result, you usually have a faster recovery. You may be able to leave the hospital a day earlier and go back to work sooner.

47) **Do I have to be asleep during the surgery?**

No. There are two major types of anesthesia that can be used for carrying out the radical prostatectomy. One is called epidural anesthesia, in which the lower abdomen and pelvis are numbed. However, you can be completely awake or can be somewhat drowsy if intravenous (IV) sedation is requested. General anesthesia also can be used for a radical prostatectomy. With this type of anesthesia you are unconscious, so a tube is placed in your throat so that a machine can breathe for you during the surgery.

48) **How much blood loss can I expect from surgery?**

The amount of blood loss can vary from one patient to the next. An average amount of blood loss is approximately 750 to 1,500 ml (between about 25 and 50 ounces). Most often, this amount of blood loss will not require a blood transfusion.

49) **What kind of scar will I have after surgery and how many stitches will I need?**

If a radical retropubic prostatectomy is performed, the scar will be vertical, from the navel to the pubic bone. If a radical perineal prostatectomy is performed, the scar will be a u-shaped semicircle between the scrotum and the anus. The number of stitches required depends upon the length of the incision. Also, there are some surgeons who place the stitches under the skin so they are not seen and don't need to be removed.

50) **What kind of erections and ejaculations will I have after surgery?**

The nerve-sparing radical prostatectomy will allow you to have erections after surgery. However, the strength of your erections will depend on your age and the strength of your erections before surgery. Younger men usually have stronger erections. However, your ejaculations will be "dry," which means little to no fluid will be released because the prostate and seminal vesicles (which make most of the seminal fluid) are removed during surgery. Sperm will still be made by the testicles, however. Also, even if you cannot have erections, it is still possible to have a sex drive and orgasms.

51) **How soon after the surgery can I have hospital visitors?**

In most hospitals, it is possible for you to have visitors upon returning from the recovery room. Usually you are quite comfortable and can visit with your immediate family and close friends.

52) **I know the hospital stay is usually between three and seven days, but can I stay longer just to be sure I am in the best shape possible when I leave the hospital?**

You should go home as soon as possible, because the longer you are hospitalized, the greater your risk for picking up an infection. The hospital is a clean place, but it is also full of people who have a lot of different diseases. Besides, you will likely recover just as fast at home.

53) **I live far from the hospital. Is it OK to fly home after I am released from the hospital or should I ride in a car?**

After undergoing radical prostatectomy or any other invasive treatment for prostate cancer, this decision should be left entirely up to you and your family. Either mode of transportation is acceptable. If going by car, we suggest stopping every 100 to 150 miles so you can walk around the car several times. This will help prevent any blood clots from forming in your legs. If you are going to fly, we suggest securing a seat with additional leg room. This will allow you to be more comfortable. Also, you should get up every hour or so and take a short walk in the aisle of the plane.

54) **Is it possible to get a woman pregnant after surgery?**

Yes. There is a procedure called "needle aspiration," in which sperm is removed from the testicles and is used for in-vitro fertilization. There is a 30 percent success rate for each attempt and the average cost is $8,500 per attempt (usually not covered by insurance).

55) **How soon can I drive, resume household chores and exercise after surgery?**

In general, it is a good idea to take it easy for two to three weeks after the procedure. After that time, it is certainly possible to drive a car (if your car has power steering) and do minor tasks around the house. With regard to strenuous exercise (playing golf, tennis or weight lifting), we would suggest waiting at least six weeks. This also goes for riding a bicycle, during which pressure is placed directly on your bottom.

56) **Can I go on vacation after surgery?**

Absolutely. Many patients do. It is a nice idea to go to your favorite location and relax as you recover from this operation.

57) **If my surgery is not successful, can I still undergo external- beam radiation therapy or some other kind of treatment?**

Yes. You can still have external-beam radiation therapy and hormonal treatment. However, since you no longer have a prostate, you are not eligible for cryosurgery or radioactive seed implants.

C

What are some of the most common questions (uncommonly asked) about experimental treatments?

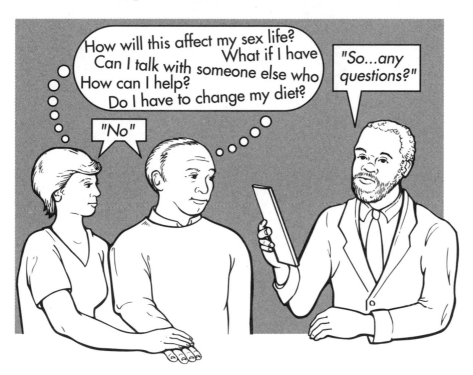

Cryosurgery

1) Do I have to change my diet, have an enema, or take any antibiotics before or after cryosurgery?

Because cryosurgery involves placing an ultrasound probe in the rectum, your doctor will most likely instruct you to have an enema in the evening before the procedure to make sure the area is clean. Also, you will be given intravenous antibiotics just prior to beginning the cryosurgical procedure. You also may need to take antibiotics for a day or two afterward.

2) **Is there anything I can do before or after cryosurgery to give myself a better outcome or a faster recovery?**

No.

3) **Can I have intercourse or ejaculate before or after cryosurgery?**

Yes, you can have sexual intercourse before cryosurgery. After the operation, as soon as you have recovered sufficiently, it is possible to again engage in sexual activities. However, you should remember that it may take as long as a year for normal erections to return.

4) **Do I have to stop drinking, smoking and eating fatty foods before or after cryosurgery?**

No. However, it is always wise to avoid these habits to maintain the best possible health.

5) **How much blood loss can I expect from cryosurgery?**

A minimal amount.

6) **What kind of scar will I have after cryosurgery and how many stitches will I need?**

There will be five very small, 1-cm incisions in the skin between the scrotum and the anus. They each will be closed with one stitch. Thus, after you are completely healed, it may be possible to notice five very, very small scars in that area.

7) **How soon can I drive, resume household chores and exercise after cryosurgery?**

While it is possible to carry out more of these activities immediately after cryosurgery than after a radical prostatectomy, you should still take it easy until you feel totally comfortable, usually at least six weeks. You should wait at least six weeks before riding a bicycle, however, to avoid putting pressure on your rear.

8) **Can I go on vacation after cryosurgery?**

Absolutely.

9) **Can I still have surgery, external-beam therapy or radiation-seed implants if the cryosurgery is not successful?**

Yes. But of the three, external-beam radiation therapy is typically easiest to perform after cryosurgery.

Radioactive-seed implants (brachytherapy)

10) **Do I have to change my diet, have an enema, or take any antibiotics before or after brachytherapy?**

Your doctor will most likely have you take an enema in the evening before the procedure to make sure the rectal area is clean. Also, the doctor will give you antibiotics through your vein just prior to beginning the implantation procedure. You also may be asked to take antibiotics for a day or two afterward.

11) **Is there anything I can do before or after brachytherapy to give myself a better outcome or a faster recovery?**

No.

12) **Can I have intercourse or ejaculate before or after brachytherapy?**

Yes. (See Question No. 3 in this section.)

13) **Do I have to stop drinking, smoking or eating fatty foods before or after brachytherapy?**

No. (See Question No. 4 in this section.)

14) **Will I receive any type of anesthesia during the procedure?**

Yes, usually spinal anesthesia, so that you will not feel anything below the waist.

15) **How much blood loss can I expect from brachytherapy?**

A minimal amount.

16) **What kind of scar will I have after brachytherapy and how many stitches will I need?**

Similar to cryosurgery, there will be five very small, 1-cm incisions in the skin between the scrotum and the anus. They each will be closed with one stitch. Thus, after you are completely healed, it may be possible to notice five very, very small scars in this area.

17) **Since I am getting radiation, is it safe for my family and friends to come near me after this procedure?**

Yes and no. Yes, family and friends can get near you, but pregnant women and children should stay at least 6 feet away for the first few months.

18) **Can I ride a bike, exercise, clean the house or drive a car after brachytherapy?**

Indeed, it is possible to carry out more of these activities immediately after brachytherapy than after a radical prostatectomy. However, you should take it easy until you feel comfortable with these different activities. As far as riding a bicycle is concerned, you should wait at least six weeks.

19) **Can I go on vacation after brachytherapy?**

Absolutely.

20) **If the treatment is not successful, can I get another seed implant? Would I be a candidate for cryosurgery, external-beam radiation therapy, radical prostatectomy or other additional treatments?**

After radioactive seed-implants, it is possible to still undergo external-beam radiation therapy and androgen-deprivation therapy. However, it is not suggested to have either cryosurgery or a radical prostatectomy. The complications of these two procedures after radioactive-seed implantation are substantial.

21) **Can I have intercourse or ejaculate before or after radioactive seed implants?**

Yes. However, you should abstain for a few days after the implant procedure just to be safe.

Medical References

Title: **"The man's cancer. Prostate cancer is reaching epidemic levels in the U.S. This is no time for squeamishness"**
Author: Jaroff, L.
Journal: *Time*
Volume: 147 (14)
Pages: 58-65
Date: April 1996

Title: **"My battle with prostate cancer"**
Author: Grove, A.
Journal: *Fortune*
Volume: No volume listed
Pages: 54-72
Date: May 1996

Title: **"The dilemmas of prostate cancer"**
Authors: Garnick, M.B.
Journal: *Scientific American*
Volume: No volume listed
Pages: 72-81
Date: April 1994

Title: **"The Prostate-Cancer Dilema"**
Authors: Mann, C.C.
Journal: *Atlantic Magazine*
Volume: No volume listed
Pages: 102-118
Date: November 1993

Title: **"The prostate puzzle"**
Authors: No author listed
Journal: *Consumer Report*
Volume: No volume listed
Pages: 1-7
Date: July 1993

Notes

11

The Many Faces of Prostate Cancer

A

Is prostate cancer a woman's disease?

B

Is prostate cancer a national epidemic?

C

Is prostate cancer a worldwide epidemic?

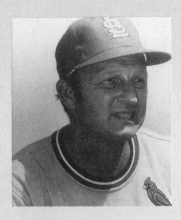

Stan Musial
Member, Baseball Hall of Fame

I played in the big leagues for 22 years and collected more than 3,600 hits, but the biggest challenge of my life has been outside the ballpark. When prostate cancer struck two years ago, I thought I was out of the game. Happily I was wrong. That's because I was diagnosed early on, during a regular checkup, and I was able to get effective treatment. I'm living proof that early detection can save your life.

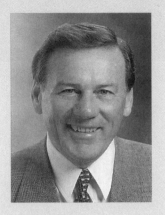

Len Dawson
Hall of Fame quarterback

Like a lot of other men, I was not exactly thrilled when my wife, Linda, told me she had scheduled a prostate-cancer screening for me. I'd had a physical about nine months before and had no symptoms of prostate disease.

It has been more than four years now since that screening revealed that I had prostate cancer. Luckily for me, my cancer was caught early enough to allow for a complete recovery. Had Linda not insisted that I keep that appointment, I might not have been so fortunate.

Routine prostate-cancer checkups are essential to early diagnosis and proper treatment — and peace of mind, not only for the man, but everyone who cares about him.

A

Is prostate cancer a woman's disease?

Women do not have prostates, and so they cannot get prostate cancer. It's that simple. Or is it?

In reality, prostate cancer is very much a woman's disease. When a man is diagnosed, the woman closest to him must not only deal with the cancer but with the variety of new roles she suddenly finds herself assuming — care giver, head of the household, therapist, patient advocate, medical researcher — the increased responsibilities are nearly limitless.

Studies done in the 1980s on patients with different types of cancer revealed that spouses have a more difficult time dealing with the diagnosis than do the patients.

But ironically, without the influence of the spouse, many men wouldn't find out about their prostate cancer in the first place. If we had a dime for every health care provider who told us about a patient whose prostate cancer wouldn't have been diagnosed or treated properly if his wife hadn't dragged him in for a checkup, we could retire tomorrow. If we had a dime for every patient who told us he could not have imagined going through the experience of prostate cancer without his spouse, we again could retire tomorrow.

A recent study out of New York City's Memorial Sloan-Kettering Cancer Center looked at the effect of prostate cancer on the man and his spouse. (see Fig. 11A) Most of the patients received hormonal therapy (55 percent), some received radiation therapy and/or surgery (28 percent), and others (18 percent) did not receive any treatment. The average age of the patients was 68 years, while the average age of the spouses was 63. The treatments and ages may have varied but the results did not: The women endured a greater overall trauma than did the actual patients. In almost all of the comparable categories, a larger percentage of women were affected than men. These categories included fatigue (being tired, needing to rest, lack of energy, feeling ill) and psychological prob-

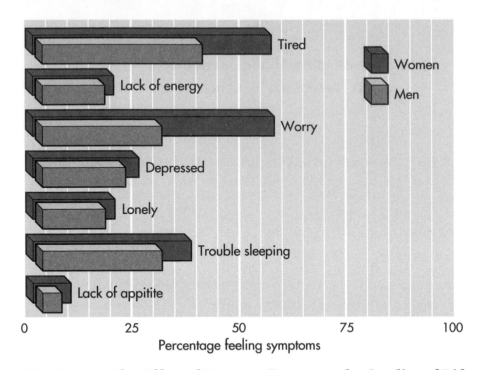

Fig. 11A — The Effect of Prostate Cancer on the Quality of Life of Men and their Spouses

lems such as being worried, depressed, tense, irritable and lonely. The women also had more problems sleeping and eating than their husbands. The authors tried to look into the possible causes for such one-sided results and felt it could not be explained completely by just gender differences. In other words, many of these women were probably being affected as much as, if not more than, the men.

Another study measured cortisol (steroid) levels in the blood of female relatives of patients who had terminal cancer. The level of cortisol in the bloodstream is an indicator of the amount of stress a person is experiencing. The higher the cortisol level, the more stress they are feeling. The age range of the women in this study was 24-72, but the results indicated increased cortisol levels and stress among women of all ages.

Finally, we are not downplaying the actual stress the man goes through when dealing with prostate cancer or even the possibility of having the disease. We realize it can be as traumatic — if not more so — for the man, and that the stress level varies on an individual basis. However, prostate cancer is also a woman's disease and we need to start recognizing this fact much more than we have in the past.

In this section you'll meet a few women who have been affected by prostate cancer and their experiences with this disease. Some of their stories are dark — even downright depressing. Some are light and hopeful. Others are a mixture of both, colored in shades of gray.

Why would we include some depressing stories in this book? The answer is simple: They represent reality. And we hope you, the reader, will never forget another reality: that behind nearly every man with prostate cancer, there's a woman suffering in her own way from the disease. Here are some of their stories:

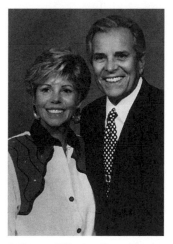

April Becker

Founder, Prostate Cancer
Communication Resource
Carefree, Ariz.

Her husband, Larry Becker, is a survivor of advanced prostate cancer

In June 1991 my husband, Larry, was diagnosed with prostate cancer following a routine PSA test. I was totally devastated and so was he. Panic stricken, we made an appointment with a urologist at the Mayo Clinic. Larry opted for a radical prostatectomy and was operated on about a month after the diagnosis. His PSA was 18 at the time. During the operation, it was discovered that the cancer had spread to the lymph nodes, so an orchiectomy (surgical removal of the testes) was performed in accordance with my husband's wishes.

Larry's current PSA is 0.1; to date, there is no sign the cancer has returned. However, as my husband is quick to note, you're only as good as the results of your last PSA test. In retrospect, we now realize how little we knew about prostate cancer five years ago or how drastically our lives would change.

The most difficult thing that I had to cope with after Larry's operation was not having anyone to talk with. I didn't know anyone who had gone through what we were experiencing. We now know that Larry was in the grips of a major depression, but at the time, neither of us realized it. Larry was also suffering from lack of energy, frustration over the loss of his potency and, even more devastating, his lack of sexual feelings, or libido. I felt confused, helpless and frustrated. I even felt guilty for feeling all of those things, because he was the one with cancer. In fact, when Larry began to avoid any physical contact with me, I thought that I had done something wrong. It took years for us to get our lives back on track because at the time, no one was properly addressing the emotional and psychological ramifications of prostate cancer.

Approximately a year after Larry's diagnosis we were invited to attend the first meeting of the Phoenix chapter of US TOO, an international prostate-cancer support group. Both Larry and I since have been extremely involved in the support-group movement.

It was during our early days as members of US TOO that I became increasingly aware of how little attention was being focused on significant others. Didn't anyone realize that women suffer from prostate cancer too? It was that first cry of indignation that later became the slogan of my efforts on behalf of women affected by prostate cancer. After hearing about a women's prostate-cancer support group in Florida, I contacted Joan Kinter, the founder of Side-By-Side, a nonprofit support group for women whose spouses, family members or close friends have prostate cancer. With Joan's blessing I organized the second chapter of this much-needed organization in the Phoenix metropolitan area. I'm happy to report that Side-By-Side has now been taken over by the American Cancer Society. Hopefully, it will become as prevalent as the support groups for men.

It has become so apparent to us that one of the major obstacles to coping with the emotional and psychological ramifications of prostate cancer is the reticence of those affected by it to talk about it. Of all the messages we would like to send to those who are impacted by this deadly disease, it is the importance of communication. Talk to each other. Talk to your family. Talk to your doctors. In today's more enlightened environment, there's absolutely no need to suffer in silence.

In early 1996, realizing the importance of this aspect of dealing with prostate cancer, Larry and I formed a nonprofit education and information corporation called the Prostate Cancer Communication Resource. Our goal is to provide programs to men, women and couples to help them improve their communication and coping skills, and to create unique programs for corporations and service organizations to increase men's awareness of the need for annual prostate checkups. We've also developed a Prostate Cancer Couples Workshop to help survivors and their loved ones better cope with the emotional and psychological problems associated with the side effects of treatment.

I won't mince words. The last five years have been a whirlwind of anger, fear, frustration, uncertainty, indifference, anxiety and depression. But out of all the turmoil has come the life-enriching experience of helping ourselves by helping others. If we could have but one wish come true, it would be to have the medical community recognize that treatment of the emotional and psychological side effects are among the most important issues facing prostate-cancer survivors and their families. And for those readers who have been diagnosed with this deadly disease, I offer three words of advice: Learn. Ask. Talk.

Read everything you can lay your hands on related to prostate cancer. Before seeing your doctor, make a written list of all the questions you want to ask him or her, and be sure to record the answers. Share your feelings with your loved ones and family. Release your emotions — don't hold back. Talking will help you to cope and help others to understand.

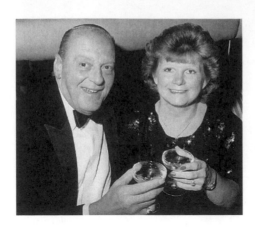

Betty Gallo

Legal assistant/prostate-cancer advocate
Succasunna, N.J.

Her husband, Congressman Dean Gallo, died of prostate cancer at age 58

In August 1991, my husband, Dean, (at the time we were not married) started to complain of a backache. I asked him repeatedly to see a doctor. Finally, a couple of months later, he saw a chiropractor. Dean continued with the chiropractor for a couple of months but was still not getting enough relief.

The chiropractor recommended that Dean see an orthopedist, who gave him a couple of cortisone shots. Dean felt a little relief but not a lot. The doctor then ordered a bone scan.

On Feb. 10, 1992, my whole life changed. I called Dean when I got home from work and he said that he needed to talk. Of course, I couldn't wait to go to his house to talk, so I asked him to please tell me what was wrong. "I have prostate cancer. My bone scan lit up like a Christmas tree," Dean said. I was stunned.

At that point I did not even know what prostate cancer was, where it was located or how serious it was.

The next day, Dean had a biopsy and a PSA blood test. The biopsy showed cancer activity and his PSA level was over 800. When Dean told me this, the first thing I did was pray.

Dean's urologist recommended an orchiectomy, an operation to remove his testes so that his body would no longer produce the male hormone testosterone, which stimulates cancer growth. I thought before we went to that extreme we should check out alternative treatments. At this time, I was not aware that Dean's condition was so far advanced that he should have survived only three to six months.

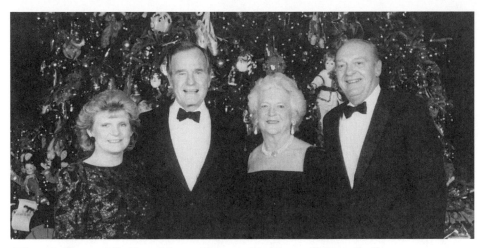

The Gallos with President George Bush and first lady
Barbara Bush.

We heard about an experimental drug treatment being offered by the National Institutes of Health that was producing good results. Dean entered the study and started on a drug called suramin, and his PSA level soon began to drop.

By January 1993 Dean's PSA was down to 3, and he said to me, "Honey, I can't believe I have cancer, because I have no pain."

At this point we had been going together for more than six years. Dean knew I really loved him, and he finally realized how much he loved me and how important I was in his life.

That April we went on a cruise to St. Martin and St. Thomas. It was the most wonderful time for both of us. This is where Dean asked me to marry him. We set the date for Sept. 17, 1994, his mother's birthday.

After that, his PSA level went up and down as he participated in several other NIH treatment protocols.

Finally, in August 1994, Dean decided to retire from Congress. By September, our wedding month, he was having some pain, so the doctors gave him an injection of strontium, a radioactive compound that is usually pretty successful in treating bone pain. Unfortunately, it did the opposite to Dean and created more pain, and he was hospitalized.

Because of the setback, we got married a week earlier than planned, on Sept. 10. The ceremony took place in the hospital chapel, and the staff prepared a wonderful reception in a conference room. Dean said to me on that day that I would never know how much he loved me. It was the happiest day of our lives.

Those two and a half years since he was diagnosed were the best years of our relationship. We were so close with our love and with the Lord. Our faith is what got us through such a devastating situation and kept us going. From the time Dean was diagnosed, the one thing he and I began to do was go to church. Dean had a very busy schedule, but he tried to make Sunday morning church a priority unless there was an obligation he just could not miss.

Dean was released from the hospital on Sept. 13. There were some tough times with the pain at home, so Dean had decided to let hospice tend to his care. I knew what bringing in hospice meant, but I told the nurse and social worker that I would not give up hope and would not accept the fact that he would die. I told them that I would do everything for Dean.

We tried different diets, vitamins and herbal teas. We had the church elders come in and pray over Dean for physical healing. We also changed doctors. The one we chose was highly recommended and believed in aggressive treatment. This made Dean and I feel better.

We started a new treatment protocol, but it had to be interrupted in October, when Dean fell and broke his shoulder and had to be admitted to the hospital.

The next couple of weeks were up and down, but I never gave up hope that something would turn this situation around.

President Bush came to New Jersey for an event honoring Dean's retirement from Congress. Unfortunately, Dean could not attend. The president also came to the hospital and saw Dean before the event, which drew nearly 1,000 people. The telephone company had hooked up a special phone line so Dean could hear the whole program from his hospital room. It was a wonderful tribute.

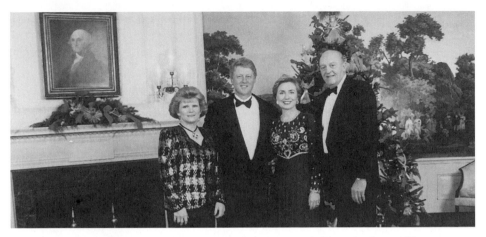

The Gallos with President Bill Clinton and first lady Hillary Rodham Clinton.

That night, Dean was put on oxygen. A few days later, a holistic nurse came to see if she could "take away his bad energy." That same night my pastor came to see him. Later, in the hospital cafeteria, I told the pastor that I had spoken with the Lord after Dean was diagnosed and the Lord had promised me he would heal him. The pastor said to me, "The Lord does not always heal physically, but spiritually."

The next three days, Dean was quiet. He didn't eat much or even watch TV. Then, on a Thursday morning, a nurses' aide called me at home and said Dean was very upset. I rushed to the hospital and Dean said to me, "Honey, I cannot do this anymore. I want to die and be with the Lord." I said, "Whatever you want, I am here for you." I told the nurses to call the rest of the family. A couple of hours later, Dean turned to me and said, "How long is this going to take?" I didn't know what to say. I wished I had a heavenly telephone so I could find out for him. It was a humorous moment in a very sad situation.

The next day, Dean was in tremendous pain. It was horrible. I just wanted him to stop suffering. The doctor raised Dean's level of morphine and gave him some Ativan, which made him semi-conscious. The last thing Dean said was, "Jesus, please take me now."

In the early morning hours of Sunday, Nov. 6, 1994, Dean's breathing became labored. The family sat and waited. Finally, at 11:25 a.m. I was sitting outside his door and the nurses' light came on. I knew something was happening. I rushed into Dean's room and looked at him as he drew his last breath. It was the most painful experience, other than my mother's death, that I had ever encountered. I knew he had died. I also knew he was at peace. I touched his body and could feel the emptiness. It was the first time I had ever touched someone after they had died. It helped me not be afraid of death.

The following days were like a blur. The funeral attendees included Dean's congressional and state colleagues, and present and past governors of New Jersey. There were about 900 people there. At the burial, Dean had a 21-gun salute, and I was presented with the flag from his coffin.

After the funeral, it was so difficult to know what to do with myself, especially having been involved in Dean's care for so long. Now there was a void.

When Dean retired from Congress, he and I were going to take on the advocacy of education, awareness and early detection of prostate cancer. Since his death I've felt the need to carry this advocacy on.

I've worked with the American Cancer Society to establish the Dean Gallo Memorial Softball Tournament. The first tournament, held in August 1995, raised more than $15,000. I have testified before the Assembly Health Committee, which designated June as Prostate Awareness Month in Dean's memory. I've written letters to the editor about the importance of early detection and awareness of prostate cancer. I have lobbied Congress, on behalf of the American Foundation for Urologic Disease, for federal funding of PSA testing and prostate-cancer education. I have testified before the New Jersey Senate Health Committee for better insurance coverage of PSA blood tests and digital-rectal exams. I am also involved in a national prostate-cancer task force and frequently speak at various functions.

Working to raise awareness of prostate cancer has truly helped me deal with the grieving process since Dean's death. Looking back, I can honestly say that I was not mad that Dean had prostate cancer. The experience actually made him a more sensitive and emotional person. The closeness and love we had was incredible. I will probably never experience that again. I do wish that he could have lived longer, but we are never in control of our destiny.

My goal is to help prevent others from suffering from prostate cancer the way Dean did by advocating the importance of early detection, awareness and education. In doing so, I know that when I leave this earth, I will have made a difference, as did my husband — and that we will again be together.

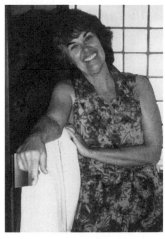

Rosemary Hamelburg

Travel agent
Braintree, Mass.

Her husband, Manny Hamelburg (whose story appears on Page 263), is a survivor of advanced prostate cancer

My name is Rosemary Hamelburg. I am 56 years old, live with my husband and best friend, Manny, spend most of my free time with my magnificent children and grandchildren, and work as a travel agent so that Manny and I can travel frequently. Today life seems precious and fragile, calm and turbulent, sweet and agonizingly painful, stable and precarious — all at the same time.

My life as I know it today began on Oct. 27, 1987, when we were told that Manny had prostate cancer. I can still remember physically backing away from the doctor, as if putting a distance between me and his impossibly crazy words could erase the fact that my 47-year-old husband had a dreaded disease that was supposed to happen only to much older men. Cancer. How can one six-letter word so completely shatter two individuals, one couple and an entire family?

After the initial shock, the running from doctor to doctor and Manny's daily radiation treatments were over, we caught our breath and looked at each other. Our special close relationship had been threatened. Manny had faced death and I had faced aloneness. Neither of us felt at all in control or any longer secure. And so we lived. We traveled and bought and went and did. We were rushing and keeping busy from early morning until late evening. We tried to live a lifetime each and every day. Gradually, with each positive checkup, I started to slow down. I felt more relaxed and finally came to believe that the cancer was a thing of the past. Our lives became more settled and normal, the way it was supposed to be.

If I thought I had been shocked and devastated in 1987, I can't begin to describe the emotions that engulfed me when, in 1992, we discovered that the cancer was again active and had metastasized to the bones. We again ran from doctor to doctor before spending nine weeks at the National Institutes of Health in Bethesda, Md., where Manny underwent experimental treatment. It was so awful being separated from my family and friends, frightened and unsure if Manny would live or die. And as if that weren't enough, it was during that time that Manny's business was liquidated, leaving us both unemployed and without any financial security.

We finally returned home, where we were surrounded by our wonderfully devoted children, extended family and friends. I recognized that my children were terribly shaken and frightened. They looked to me for support. I saw these adults as they were when they were kids, looking to Mom to make it all better. I could not make it better. I could not help them. I felt directionless and lost. I drifted from day to day, jumped at the slightest upset and was unable to concentrate or sleep. I just could not get on with the process of living.

To my credit, I at least knew that I was unable to make progress by myself. I sought professional help. I took advantage of individual as well as couple, family and group therapy. I accepted help from medication. I went with Manny to all of his support groups. I hated wasting this precious time Manny and I had together by panicking about what the future would bring.

Gradually I came to realize that my needs were very different from Manny's. His support groups were actually harmful to me because I found I was stifling my thoughts and wants if they differed from those that he expressed. I was trying to protect him. I finally understood that I couldn't help Manny until I began to help myself. So I went to travel school, became an agent and got a job. It felt positive to take action instead of just drifting along.

In the last year I, like my husband, have taken advantage of the Wellness Community. I attend weekly meetings for family members of cancer patients. We share common feelings and needs, and give and get support from each other. I almost never miss a session. These days, I look at Manny and just marvel at his strength, confidence, positive attitude and sense of fulfillment. I am jealous of his newly found peace of mind. I feel anything but peaceful. My once organized, capable, dependable qualities seem to have been replaced with inner turmoil and confusion. I feel very fragile. I often feel out of control.

I struggle with my desire to retire and spend more time with Manny, while at the same time I want the money and travel experience my job provides. I miss the ability to lean and depend on Manny for solid support. I see him struggling to maintain the contentment that he has achieved. I love Manny. I treasure each day and each experience we share. I hate that his cancer has spoiled our "happily ever after." I am trying very hard to accept what we have been given and to appreciate what we do have for however long we are together.

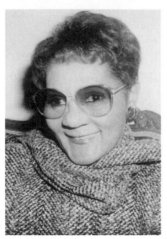

Anna C. Harris

Retired Red Cross executive
Silver Spring, Md.

Her husband, Harry Harris (whose story appears on Page 266), was diagnosed with prostate cancer at age 69

That momentous drive down to South Carolina remains vivid in my mind. I knew that there was more to it than a mere bladder full of Coke.

My husband, Harry, thought his problem was attributed to excessive Coke drinking when he pulled over on the shoulder of I-95 to empty his bladder. He had such a sudden and compelling need, he could not even contemplate reaching the next comfort station; he had to go that instant or face an even greater embarrassment! Embarrassed? Humiliated? Mild words! Harry, a tall, stately man — a retired lieutenant colonel with the U.S. Army who obeys the law to a "T" — was distressed and confused. Distressed because he had been forced to break the law (one isn't supposed to pull over and do that) and confused because he did not understand what was happening to him. For a man always in command and in control of himself, what on earth could have precipitated this sudden onrush and urgent need to urinate? He had no answer and apologized profusely. I sensed a feeling of helplessness and bewilderment in his tone as he offered apologies and rationalizations. I could sense that he wanted to turn around and return home, but he was thinking about me and the long-planned trip, the disappointment, and bravely continued the journey. The same thing happened later in the trip. Harry was devastated. He became meek, withdrawn and even more bewildered.

During our vacation, he cut back on his consumption of Coke and drank very little water. The sudden and compelling need to urinate did not recur. My husband is a man of action when involved with others. One has only to express a desire and it is done. But when it comes to taking care of his own affairs, I'd rank him among the top procrastinators. He did not go to see the doctor upon our return, as he had promised. Months went by, and I heard no further complaints. I did, however, notice frequent, hurried visits to the bathroom day and night.

One September morning in 1991, he walked out of the bathroom and approached me with a look on his face I had never seen before. "Look, I passed blood in my urine," he said. There was grave concern in his voice as he assured me that he was free of any disease, that he had done nothing to cause this. My heart went out to him that moment, and I wanted to assure him that I would stand by him in all kinds of weather — in sickness and in health. But instead, I took on the motherly role and said, "OK, no more putting off, you have to go see the doctor today. This is a clear indication that something is wrong somewhere and has to be taken care of right away." I offered to accompany him to the hospital, but he declined and went alone.

"The doctor says it is nothing serious, that I am OK. Unless it happens again, not to worry," Harry reported to our profound mutual relief. Cranberry juice replaced the Coke in the refrigerator and I urged him to drink as much of it as possible to flush out the bladder. The blood traces dissipated and everything went back to normal.

Months passed. Then, one day, when Harry was at the barber shop, he saw an article about prostate cancer in *Stripe*, a weekly publication of the Walter Reed Army Medical Center. He said he had experienced almost all of the symptoms mentioned in the article, from difficult urination to blood in the urine. In fact, he said he had experienced some of these symptoms as far back as 1964, during his U.S. Special Forces tour of duty in Vietnam. He'd attributed the symptoms to the fact that he refrained from drinking water — only canned beverages (he's a teetotaler) and iced tea.

He decided right then and there to get a prostate examination. The doctor referred him to a urologist who, after a series of additional tests, pronounced that Harry had prostate cancer.

My husband, who had never complained about a headache, a toothache, a stomachache, a backache, who had never run a temperature, had CANCER. The thought of death flashed through my mind but faded away as quickly as it had come. Never again have I thought of him dying from prostate cancer. My primary concern was that he live a healthy, meaningful and quality life.

Luckily, the doctor didn't think Harry's cancer had spread, so he had a variety of treatment options, from watchful waiting to prostate-removal surgery to radiation therapy to cryosurgery. We read all the literature and went through the process of elimination. Harry decided to use the Army modus operandi: mean, quick and dirty. Surgery, he said, was the way to go: mean, quick and dirty. Recovery would be a one-time shot — in and out of the hospital, no traveling back and forth for treatment. I supported his decision, the doctor was informed and a surgery date was set.

Recovery went as well as expected both in the hospital and at home. Within six weeks he was back behind the wheel, driving himself to the hospital and doing little chores around the house. Recovery came very rapidly for him, and soon the distance of his daily walks increased. He played golf three months after surgery and resumed going to church services. Today he is not on any medication or treatment and continues to bring home good news from his semi-annual follow-up appointments with the urologist.

Today, nearly five years after surgery, I would say Harry's recovery, comparatively speaking, is about 90 percent complete. I am so glad to have him with me, and well. Thanks to God and Walter Reed Army Medical Center's team of professionals, he's just fine!

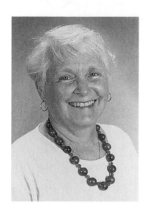

Peg Howard, M.A., R.N.

Oncology nurse
Annapolis, Md.

A support-group leader whose father died of prostate cancer

In October 1991, the third US TOO prostate-cancer support group met at George Washington University in Washington, D.C. About 30 men and women gathered. One man in particular was very angry that I, a woman, was facilitating and coordinating this group. He complained that I didn't have a prostate and therefore could not know what it was like to suffer from this disease. He did not know that my dad had died a very miserable death from prostate cancer in 1975 and I had vowed to work with this population in the future. He did not know that I, as an oncology-certified nurse, had worked with men and their families who were dealing with all stages of prostate cancer. He did not know I had a master's degree in counseling. He did not know that I had a husband, two sons, seven sons-in-law and three brothers, all who had prostates, all who I cared about. But most of all, he did not know that the other men and women who were there trusted me, wanted me there, did not agree with him and were embarrassed by his behavior.

In the years since our group began, I can say that I have learned more about prostate cancer, its diagnosis, treatment options, and ongoing research than I would ever have known otherwise. The importance of the group process in decision-making was and continues to be a powerful experience. We meet every month, usually with a guest speaker (a physician, nurse, nutritionist, sex therapist or a prostate-cancer survivor with a special message to share). We then have a sharing/caring session, which is usually the light of the day. The men and women have come to be like a family. Some of the men have been with the group from the beginning, attending almost every month; others come and go as they feel the need to attend. We have had several deaths, none of which have been sudden, but all nevertheless grieved by the group.

I have had the opportunity to talk with experts on prostate cancer from all over the country, participate in national prostate-cancer education programs and write articles for journals. However, the most rewarding and touching experience has been the support and love I received from the group when I was diagnosed with breast cancer. They were there for me as they are for each other.

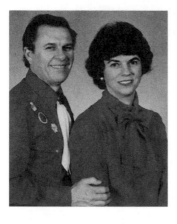

Betty Jones
Housewife
Baltimore, Md.

Her husband, Brandt Jones, died of prostate cancer at age 56

Prostate cancer. The words hit me like a knife in my gut. I looked at my husband Brandt. His face showed the same shock and disbelief that I felt. One of us asked the doctor how bad it was. I remember him saying on a scale of one to 10, 10 being the worst, my husband was a nine. I learned later that that was his Gleason score.

Prostate; I searched my brain. I knew it was a small male organ somewhere in the pelvic region, but I wasn't too sure of its function. Little did I know as Brandt and I walked out of the urologist's office our lives had just made a 180-degree turn. The next 22 months were consumed with doctor visits, treatments, operations, medicine and horror. Shock, denial, anger at God, bargaining with God, and the never-ending research, research and more research. I truly believe I became as knowledgeable as the men and women in white who treated, operated on and cared for Brandt.

Brandt was too young, only 54 years old. I was too young, only 49. This was supposed to be an old man's disease. Not so! I met one man with prostate cancer who was just 29. We joined US TOO support groups, three of them. We located the best doctors in the field. We talked to anyone who knew anything about the disease. I spent hours in medical libraries poring over anything written about prostate cancer, a publication in one hand and a medical dictionary in the other. And what was the end result? Twenty-two months

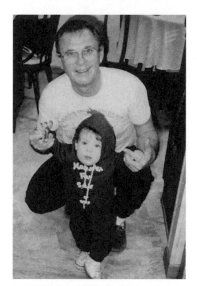

The late Brandt Jones with his grandson Nicholas David Eber.

later, after 34 years of a wonderful marriage that should have lasted twice that long, Brandt was dead.

From that first day in the doctor's office he went steadily downhill. He lost every battle and finally the war. I won't go into all the clinical details — these are covered elsewhere in this book. I'll just mention some of our feelings and the ways we dealt with them.

In the beginning, Brandt was a healthy, active man. Retired from the Navy, he had a good second job, was a SCUBA instructor, a cross-country and downhill skier, a 33-degree Mason, an advanced square dancer and a canoeist.

His first PSA test (a 14) picked up the cancer. His yearly physicals, which always included a digital-rectal exam, never found the tumor because it was growing on the far side of his prostate.

Then the treatments, procedures, tests and medicine began. Before it was all over he had suffered through prostate and lymph-node biopsies, many bone scans, a radical prostatectomy, several bladder constrictions, four urethral dilations, several CAT scans, a sonogram, a 3-D bone scan, blood tests, urine tests, spine X-rays, four spine biopsies, a splenectomy and countless catheterizations. He also suffered from lymphedema (fluid buildup) from the chest down and had to wear support stockings on his legs. He made many trips to the National Institutes of Health to discuss experimental treatments like suramin, chemotherapy and medicine, medicine and more medicine.

During the months he was dying, his cancer spread to his spine, liver and lungs. His left kidney ceased to function and a large blood clot formed in one thigh. There was nausea, vomiting and sweating. There was pain in his legs, back and abdomen. He was constipated. His mouth was dry. His liver and throat were swollen. He was in a wheelchair. His speech was slurred. His skin was yellow. His legs oozed with fluid and burned like they were on fire. It was hard for him to breathe, and he spit up phlegm. His eyes became dry and itchy. He lost bowel and bladder control. He lost his hair. His voice became hoarse and then he lost that, too. Most of his vision was gone — what was left was double, so he wore a patch over one eye. He alternated between sleepiness and restlessness. He drooled. He was so weak he couldn't move. He hallucinated.

His PSA was over 5,000.

Finally it ended. Cradled in his mother's arms, at 8:30 p.m. Sunday, Oct. 30, 1994, he died.

How did he cope with all of this? Complete denial. Somewhere early on he was told that some men with advanced prostate cancer live 15 years. He grabbed onto this time frame and made it his lifeline. He wanted to live. He had worked so hard to be able to retire at 55 and live life to the fullest — to travel, to enjoy his grandsons, to serve his family and community. He had worked hard for it.

Let me give you an example of his complete denial. Five days before he died he asked me to have a ring guard put on his wedding band because he was so thin it kept falling off his finger. The jeweler, (a friend who knew about prostate cancer) re-sized the ring instead of putting on the ring guard, but charged me only the lower price of the guard. Later when Brandt put the ring on, which fit perfectly, he said it was nice of the jeweler to do this so cheaply, but what was he going to do with his ring, which was now so small, when he gained his weight back?

How did I cope? Every waking moment was spent caring for him and doing research. There had to be a way to save him. God knows how I tried. I even injected six needles with saline solution into my own thigh to learn how to give injections so I could bring him home from the hospital. Knowing he was dying didn't prepare me for the intense grief and what it was like to suddenly be living completely alone.

My future was wiped out. I had to face the unknown. I was scared. I hated being alone. Brandt always did all the home and car repair. He cared for the yard and garden. No more. Now it's up to me. I don't know how. I can't do it all. So many thank you notes to write, so many people visiting. So much house cleaning to catch up on. A year's worth of magazines and newspapers I haven't read. Mail, financial decisions, loss of income, loneliness, no companion, no best friend, no lover. Long, lonely evenings, days, weekends.

Widow — it's a word for old women. How can it be me? I'm only 51.

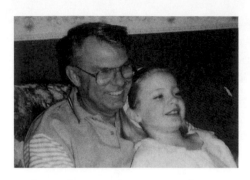

Jennifer Koontz
Age 9
Anchorage, Alaska

Her grandfather, Donald
Costley, was diagnosed with
localized prostate cancer at
age 54

I do not understand cancer,
but I saw what it did to my
family. Everyone was very sad.
I was sad because grandpa
had to have surgery and mom
had to leave us to be with
him.
I worried about grandpa everyday
that he was gone. After surgery
grandpa showed me his scares.
They looked like they hurt.
He told me it would be a long
time before he could lift me
up.
It has been a year since
then and grandpa lifts me
up into his arms alot. It is
now that I relize how important
it was for grandpa to have
surgery, because today I still
have a grandpa.
I am thankful that grandpa
found his cancer before he got
real sick. I hope that if my dad
or brother ever get prostate cancer
they will find it before they get
sick.
I hope everyone knows how
important it is to see a
doctor not only when your
sick but also to keep you
well.
         Jennifer Koontz

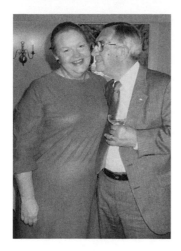

Donna J. Suwall
*Aviation teacher and
prostate-cancer advocate
Baltimore, Md.*

*Her husband, Bruno Suwall, died of
prostate cancer at age 83*

They all lied. The cancer experts, the
internists, the surgeons, the nurses, all the
printed material. They all lied.

They said prostate cancer was a man's disease. They said it was possibly hereditary,
but it was not contagious. Well, if that's true, why is it that when
my husband was diagnosed with this disease in his body, I con-
tracted it too? It's true, I did not get prostate cancer in my physical
body. Instead it lodged itself in my heart and in my soul and was to
rule my life from that day forward.

You see, by the time Bruno's cancer was discovered, it had spread
outside of his prostate gland. The doctor sat there telling us it was
inoperable, incurable and lots of other things. It's funny, but the
words that were coming out of the doctor's mouth we didn't hear,
but we could hear very clearly those words that weren't being said:
Bruno was going to die.

It was at that moment that HIS prostate cancer became MY
prostate cancer too.

I have come to know and live the full truth about prostate cancer,
which is that it is also a woman's disease. It is the woman who usually encourages the man to get the examinations. It is the woman
who becomes the main support person when prostate cancer is
diagnosed. If it is not curable, it is the woman who becomes the care
giver. And worst of all, it is the woman who has to learn to live
with the horrible pain and make a whole new life for herself when
the man she loves dies of this disease.

It has been three and a half years now since my husband died OF
prostate cancer, not WITH it. Bruno was 76 years old when his

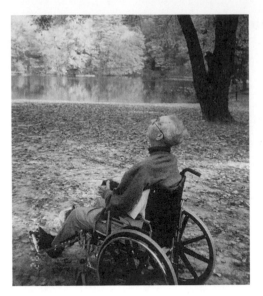

Bruno Suwall several months before he died.

cancer was diagnosed. We were told that at his age, the cancer usually spreads slowly and he probably would die with it, not of it. That proved to be untrue.

At the time of diagnosis, we had two options: radiation or watchful waiting. After much research, I learned that at his stage of the disease, the life span was usually seven to 10 years, no matter which route you chose, so we opted for watchful waiting. The year was 1983, and the sad thing is that all of this could have been prevented had the simple PSA blood test been regularly used and his cancer found before it escaped his prostate gland to become a death sentence.

Fortunately, Unfortunately is the title of a book I read to young children. Those words so well describe our battle with prostate cancer. Fortunately, we had seven good years after Bruno's diagnosis. He continued to bowl, do all the yard work, manage property we own, and travel. In 1989 we were in Italy climbing Mt. Vesuvius and he was the first to the top, even though I was much his junior in age. During those years, he was having regular PSA tests, and bone scans, and things seemed to be fine. I must admit that I was living with fear all the time, knowing there was a WHEN coming, and hoping and praying it wouldn't. Unfortunately, it came in the fall of 1990. All hell broke loose and for the next two years, terror became my constant companion. "Oh, God, please help him; please don't let him die" became my mantra.

We quickly found out how devious prostate cancer can be. Instead of going into the bones, which is the way it usually travels, tumors had been growing in Bruno's abdomen the past seven years. They created all kinds of blockages that led to one trauma after another for us until the end of his days.

All of 1991 and 1992 Bruno and I spent in and out of the hospital. He needed emergency surgery to get kidney tubes and colostomies. He needed treatment for severe infections and dehydration. No matter why we were there, I was always filled with terror: Would this be the time that he dies?

Along with this, I found I many times had to do battle with hospital staff who were incredibly insensitive to my husband's physical and emotional needs. I still cringe inside when I remember some of the unnecessary pain and discomfort he endured. I stayed with him 24 hours a day for his emotional well-being as well as his protection, and also because I wanted to be with him.

I thank God for all our friends who were so supportive during all those trials. I could never have done it without them. And I can never say enough thank-you's to all the physicians, nurses and staff at Greater Baltimore Medical Center who were so caring and worked so hard to make this struggle as easy as possible for both of us. I will forever be in their debt.

My inspiration through all this was Bruno and the heroic way he fought this battle. The only complaint I heard from this gentle man during these horrible times was made a month before he died, on Thanksgiving Day. He woke that morning and instead of saying his usual words, "Good morning, Dear, I love you," he just looked at me and said, "I know there are a lot of people in the world worse off than me, but I can't think about them right now." He went back to sleep. I sat with a broken heart and cried while I wrote our Christmas cards, knowing it would be the last time I would sign them "Donna and Bruno."

At that time I thought I was doing the hardest thing I would ever have to do — watch this man I loved more than life itself lose his vitality, slowly lose his mobility, watch him endure all the medical traumas and feel myself being forever exhausted physically and emotionally. I thought this was the hardest thing God would ever ask of me until Bruno died on Dec. 26, 1992.

It's now four years later and I can honestly say that THIS is the hardest job — learning to live and care again after his death; putting a whole new life together. The pain that consumed me when he died can only be described as a personal holocaust. My journey through this part of the "valley of death" is another story.

Bruno traveled his "valley of death" in his usual style — with incredible patience, charm, gentleness of spirit and a dry sense of humor. A week and a half before he died, he was so ill he couldn't keep his eyes open. His hospital bed was in the middle of the living room and I was walking around putting up holly for Christmas, trying to add some sense of normalcy to our days. I had put on several Christmas music tapes and really wasn't paying much attention to them. As I neared his bed he opened his eyes and said quietly, "I'm going to shoot that damn partridge!"

Had I known his family had a history of prostate cancer and had the PSA test been used as part of regular exams in 1983, I know Bruno would still be with me. He was an extremely healthy, vital man. My final gift to him is to try and spread the word about early detection and regular exams. I take every opportunity to do that — sometimes even to strangers. I teach aviation courses at a local community college and the first night of class I give my brief prostate-cancer lecture to this captive audience:

"EARLY DETECTION IS THE ONLY SURE WAY TO SAVE A LIFE! The death rate from this disease is expected to rise greatly in coming years. Save a life! Spread the word!"

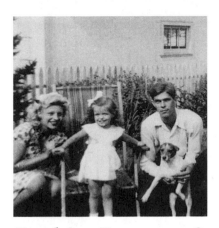

Daryl Ann Tesar, at age 2, with her mother and father (c. 1947).

Daryl Ann Tesar
Geneologist
Frankfort, Ill.

She lost her father, Arthur Carr, and both grandfathers to prostate cancer

In 1991, my mom and dad visited my brother in Atlanta and they all came down with the flu. My dad also started having pain in his upper back and breastbone. Everyone else seemed to recover, but he didn't, so he kept taking over-the-counter flu medication. You aren't supposed to take this flu medication if you have an enlarged prostate, but my dad had no idea his prostate was enlarged.

My dad was hesitant about going to the doctor. He was scared. His niece had died earlier in the year and her husband had died two years before. He said he was waiting for my son Brian to complete his medical training so he could be his doctor, as Brian was a fourth-year medical student at the time who had expressed that he might like to become a surgeon. Brian inherited his great mechanical abilities from my dad, who could fix anything.

In February 1992, my son examined my dad and he found him to have an irregular heartbeat. He told him to go to the doctor immediately. I drove my parents to the doctor, who confirmed my son's observation. He told my dad that he had to be hospitalized immediately. My dad was reluctant to do this but he did. He was a strong but sensitive man, and this was the first time I saw him cry; he was afraid that he would never leave the hospital.

My dad spent a month in the hospital, where he received a small amount of oxygen for his heart. On the second day of his hospitalization, he was discovered to have a prostate problem. At the end of the week his PSA results came back. His PSA was 600. The urologist felt that this was causing his heart problem. He recommended that his testicles be removed. The day before the operation, the results of my dad's bone scan came back. He had metastasis from head to toe. After the operation, he required blood transfusions and was delirious from the narcotics.

He had a difficult time with pain management and he was barely eating; this did not help. But then again, no one likes hospital food.

On March 10, my dad celebrated his 70th birthday. Two days later he went into renal failure. Early the next morning, he was put into intensive care.

He was also examined by a psychiatrist. Referring to his orchiectomy, he told the doctor that he had had an operation that transformed him into a female. My dad had a great sense of humor and this was his way of coping. The doctor found him to be of sound mind but in unbearable pain, despite radiation treatments to his upper spine.

At times it was difficult to communicate with some of the doctors, so I had my son Brian speak to them. I realized later that this was difficult for him, since because of his medical training, he knew exactly what was happening to his grandfather.

All my dad talked about is what would my mom do without him. I promised him he would be able to go home. On the day he left the hospital, he was 50 pounds lighter and his PSA was 143. He had appointments set up to see the doctors in two weeks. My dad needed oxygen and a hospital bed at home. The whole family was caring for him.

My dad asked me if he could go to Disney World. I wish that I could have taken him there. I knew this was his way of letting me know that he was dying.

One day I noticed my dad's legs were like ice. My son examined him and found him to be in congestive heart failure. An ambulance was called to transfer him to a hospital. My dad was anxious to go, because he now had to urinate and he couldn't; he was never on a catheter at home. When the ambulance arrived they moved my dad to the gurney and all the color drained from his face. They applied life support and called for a better-equipped ambulance. I knew he was dying. I was very upset because I had tried my best to help my dad. I only wish that I had helped sooner.

My dad was pronounced dead on April 4, 1992. He had looked forward to being a great-grandfather. He was looking forward to seeing Brian graduate from medical school in May. Instead, he was buried on April 7, 1992.

While my dad was ill, I requested information from the American Cancer Society and the prostate-cancer support group US TOO, which was looking for people to submit designs for a Prostate Awareness Pin. I created a design and sent if off. A few months later, Brooke Moran from the American Foundation for Urologic Disease called to let me know that my design had been chosen. I was so happy — what a great tribute to my dad and what a great way to make people aware of this awful disease that many people are afraid to speak about.

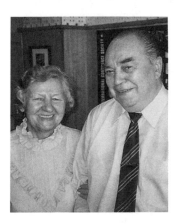

Maria Zhidovinov

Housewife
Moscow, Russia

Her husband, Vladimir Zhidovinov, is a survivor of advanced prostate cancer

My husband, Vladimir, first began to complain of urinary discomfort several years ago, and we decided it must be connected with his age and the hypertension from which he has long suffered. However, the symptoms only grew worse, and my husband had episodes of urinary retention. We decided to see a doctor. At that time, unfortunately, we knew little about the prostate gland and the necessity for men over 40 years of age to occasionally see a urologist.

An analysis of his PSA showed an increase in his level of up to 49 ng/ml. We decided to consult at Moscow's leading hospital. After additional tests and a biopsy of the prostate, it became clear that the cancer had grown to the point where one could not count on a complete removal of the tumor. My husband began treatment with combined hormonal therapy.

Taking into account his continuing problem with urination, it was suggested that my husband have a transurethral resection of the prostate and an orchiectomy, and that he continue traditional therapy with antiandrogen drugs.

It was terribly difficult at this time to learn about my husband's illness and have to decide on this operation, as he had had three heart attacks, a stroke, and suffered from hypertension, as mentioned above.

The operation went well, after which my husband's normal urinary function was restored. He continues hormonal therapy today. His PSA levels are now close to zero and it is now two years that my husband has lived with this illness. I would say that he feels quite well.

I tried to support my husband throughout this ordeal, as we have no children and it's just the two of us together in this world. Probably everyone dreams about a peaceful retirement after a life of work. Having lived together for 42 years, finding myself alone would have been a tragedy for me, the end of my existence. Two years ago it seemed like my life had come to an end. Now I try to create an atmosphere of happiness in the family and avoid talk of my husband's illness, as this can spoil our mood.

Unfortunately, at the time of my husband's diagnosis, we did not know others in a similar situation; now, however, the hospital is setting up a support group for those suffering from prostate cancer. We hope to discover new friends and have the opportunity for closer contact with each other. We have no experience with such a support group, and perhaps it will turn out that we won't want to discuss such a personal problem with strangers, but it is certainly worth a try.

Once the word cancer sounded like a death sentence. It was felt that a person suffering from this disease had only a few weeks or months to live. We hope that in the case of my husband's prostate cancer that this period will be considerably longer, that there will be more time for my husband and I to enjoy our retirement years together. We wish this all the more so because our love has remained — a love that has helped us all these years together.

B

Is prostate cancer a national epidemic?

The word "epidemic" clearly has many definitions, but the most common one is probably a disease that occurs in excess of what is expected normally. It is estimated that in the next decade, three out of every four men (75 percent) diagnosed with prostate cancer will have localized disease. In the next three years, more than 1 million men in the United States will be diagnosed with prostate cancer, and some 100,000 men will die of it. Clearly, we have a national epidemic here (see Fig.11B).

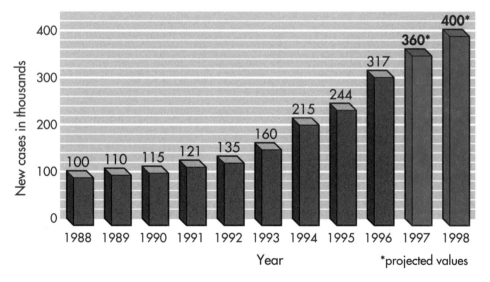

Fig. 11B — The steady increase in prostate-cancer cases in the United States makes this disease an epidemic of the past, present, and future.

Below are a few personal accounts of prostate cancer from men across the United States. Their ages and treatments may vary, but their messages are consistent: one can not only live — but live well — after a diagnosis of prostate cancer.

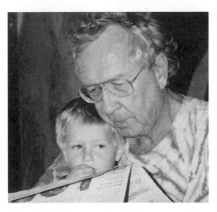

Ed DeHart with his grand-son Russell.

Ed DeHart

Semi-retired consultant
Coconut Grove, Fla.

Diagnosed with localized prostate cancer at age 69

When they told me I had prostate cancer, I was surprised. I'd already had my share of malignancies — lung cancer, skin cancer twice. I was depressed. I thought I knew how Job felt.

Prostate cancer turned out to be much harder to deal with than lung cancer.

Nine years ago, after my doctor found suspicious spots on my lung X-ray, I asked him what my options were. "Cut it out," he said.

With prostate cancer, it seems, you play multiple choice. You can cut it out, radiate it, freeze it, heat it, drug it, shoot it, cut off its food supply or ignore it. Each of these options has its pros and cons, staunch advocates (including zealots and outright evangelists) and strong critics. Naturally, they tend to advocate what they sell; the surgeons promote surgery, the radiation people promote radiation. The trouble is, it's very hard to find a dispassionate thinker. And therein lies my tale.

My internist suggested I consider radioactive-seed implants, which he felt made sense for older men. I went to see the urologist he recommended. He said surgery would be better than radiation. When asked about potency, he observed that with surgery my chances of retaining potency were probably 50-50, less with radiation. Then he tried to reassure me with talk about penile implants and injections to restore potency. "What about watchful waiting?" I asked. There was a "48-percent" chance I'd be dead in 10 years, he said. It was all happening too fast.

My objective, I decided, would be to maintain my present comfortable lifestyle for as long as possible, even at the expense of a couple more years at the end of my life.

Having made the fundamental decision — that quality was more important than length of life — the question seemed easier. Now I had a standard to measure the options against. When I told my children, I said I would beat this cancer, too. I was not going to let it change my life. I'd make appointments for tests and doctors in the mornings so I could go sailing as usual in the afternoons. In fact, my appointments and my study took over my life for the next two months.

The floor of my den was covered with papers and folders, and my phone bill was rising. There was room for little else in my life. The debate and difference of opinion reminded me of what a famed editorial writer once told me: "The facts are rarely clear cut. Usually it's like 55-45 or 51-49. But who's going to pay attention if you write a wishy-washy editorial? So we gather all our facts and make it sound like nine to one."

I knew that doctors are intimidating, even for a tough, intelligent "survivor" like me — a man who's tilted lances with lawyers, businessmen, consumer activists, regulators, legislators, scientists and media people. Most doctors don't seem to understand this. Or, maybe they like it that way. They know more than you do. They use words they understand and you often do not. They talk too fast. They're usually in a hurry. They're just working, and they don't have the cancer. That gives them a big advantage and makes it hard for a patient to think clearly in the doctor's office, much less remember what was said. I decided I would tape all future discussions. Despite the surprise, nobody objected. (One even helped me figure out how to operate my new recorder.)

My first decision, easily reached, had involved quality of life vs. lifestyle. That meant ruling out both surgery and external radiation, it seemed. Surgery would mean almost certain impotence, perhaps rectal problems and incontinence. A surgeon who offered the nerve-sparing approach to prostatectomy wouldn't even consider me in view of my age, 69. Others had said the nerve-sparing technique would not work with cancer in both lobes. And besides, I didn't like the thought of going through major surgery again, with its risks and long recovery period.

External radiation seemed about as good as surgery, based on 10-year survival data, but the side effects also seemed worrisome, including impotence, rectal problems and incontinence.

Surgery and external radiation also presented the most troublesome opportunities for the doctors, technicians or nurses to make a serious mistake. Rule No. 1 — based on my own experience and that of friends — was to stay out of the hospital. Five days of radiation a week for seven weeks presents 35 opportunities for a sleepy or sloppy technician to radiate the wrong part.

"Watchful waiting" seemed too risky, in my case, according to each of the doctors I consulted. That was also my judgment based on my reading.

I also considered cryosurgery, but I found out that impotence and rectal problems also were fairly likely. It sounded too experimental, with a paucity of hard data. Still, I wondered if this might be the wave of the future.

By now I was exhausted with reading, phoning and talking. A friend reminded me that a little knowledge can be dangerous. But, as I tried to explain to a couple of skeptical doctors, "This is the way I've lived my life. I try to find out what there is to know before I make important decisions." Sometimes, this makes me a pain in the tail.

In the middle of all this, I got a special notice from AT&T. My phone bill was much higher than normal and they wanted me to know it. This irritated me and I called. "Are you worried?" I asked. "No," she replied. "We just wanted you to know."

Also, I noted, the few people who knew about my problem had begun saying "How *are* you?" instead of "Howareya?" Years earlier, I'd learned that people assume cancer patients are going to die. This can be a real drag. When people believe they are supposed to die, they often do.

I traveled across the state to see a highly recommended urologist who does seed implants as well as surgery. (With one exception, each of the urologists I visited said they, too, could do seed implants, even while recommending surgery.) While his office staff was "patient unfriendly," he was rather impressive. I decided to tell him nothing about what others had recommended. He felt seeds would do the job standing alone, although he first suggested surgery as the best cure because, he said, "my training is in surgery."

By this time, I'd been examined by seven doctors, each of whom performed a digital exam first. "If you don't stick your finger in first, you'll put your foot in it," one of them explained. I talked with another dozen or so and queried more than 30 patients. Most of the doctors focused on length of life rather than quality. Younger white-coated men asked me impertinent questions: "Are you still active? Are you still having sex?" as though sex suddenly stopped with older men. All this reminded me of the days after lung surgery when young doctors balked at giving me enough morphine to relieve my pain for fear that I would become a drug addict (despite much research to the contrary and my lifetime of resisting drugs).

By then, I still had appointments scheduled with two more seed implant doctors. One doctor's office called after reviewing my papers. I would need weeks of external radiation first, his nurse told me. I asked if I could talk to him, to review his rationale. Her reply was frosty. "When you come out here for your appointment, in a couple of weeks, you'll have plenty of time," she said. What I heard was another two or three months of waiting, more reading, weeks of internal radiation. Well, I'd had about enough.

I reviewed my notes, listened to my tapes, talked to a friend, my shrink, my kids, and ran through the options. I listed the pros and cons. Then, I knew what to do.

My decision to choose seed radiation, initially recommended by my internist, was based in part on its relative simplicity — it's an out-patient procedure. I could probably go sailing the next day, though not bike riding. The "cure" rate seemed about as good as either surgery or external radiation out to about eight years, after which the data become meager.

The next day, I called a radiation oncologist whose long experience with implants and willingness to answer my questions had been persuasive.

"Let's schedule an appointment. I want to get this over with," I said.

It was nearly five months since my first high PSA score, about six weeks since the biopsy.

The big event itself was a snap. Afterwards, I could see the doctor's smiling face over me. "Everything went fine," he said. "How many seeds?" I asked. "Sixty-five," he replied.

Later, in the recovery room, my legs felt like lead weights. No movement. "You'll stay here until you can move your toes," the nurse said.

It was an easy, painless procedure. In one day, out the next. I stayed overnight because the procedure took place late in the day, an "add-on." Aside from the urge to pee, I felt great, comfortable with my decision.

Was it the right one? Time will tell.

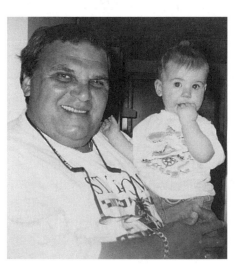

Manny Hamelburg and his granddaughter, Alexa.

Manny Hamelburg

Retired businessman
Braintree, Mass.

Diagnosed with prostate cancer at age 47

They say that if a man lives more than three years with metastatic prostate cancer he is a miracle. I am a miracle. Now, nine years after my original diagnosis and four years since metastasis, my PSA is just above 0.1, and my back pain and "hot spots" are gone. I expect to continue my miracle for many years to come.

Rosemary and I have five children; three are married. We also have four wonderful grandchildren. Now I change more diapers in a few days than I did the entire time our five children were babies. I am the world's proudest baby sitter. My family is my main motivator. My loved ones are the reason I want to go on living. They all tease me now, saying that I am obsessed with support groups and conversations with other survivors.

Support groups have been the backbone of my remarkable recovery. They provide a place to give and take emotionally, to learn the latest news related to prostate cancer, and to be able to reach out and help so many while helping myself. When I began attending meetings in January 1993, all the groups I went to stressed problems facing newly diagnosed men. But I had had a recurrence, metastatic disease. These meetings left me feeling angry, ignored by the agenda — and afraid to frighten newly diagnosed men with my personal history. As a result I, along with a few other men in similar circumstances, started a spinoff support group for survivors with advanced prostate cancer and their loved ones. We have been meeting monthly for nearly three years. The meetings vary from tearful sharing of fears and personal experiences with impotence, incontinence, pain and the "in your face" presence of death to evenings full of humor, jokes and funny anecdotes. We believe in support and openness and the strength and love we receive when we risk and help others through their tough times. I'm very proud of my part in the advanced-prostate-cancer support movement, and I have been involved in starting up new advanced groups in Boston and other areas.

It's not always positive — when a member dies of prostate cancer we all hurt. We all identify with our own vulnerability. But I believe that the pain makes me more determined to strengthen my immune system and defeat prostate cancer. I believe in the mind/body connection. I read everything I can get my hands on regarding prostate cancer, as well as books and articles related to the subject.

Talking on the phone to prostate-cancer survivors takes up a large chunk of my leisure time. I actually have business cards that say "Prostate Cancer Support Network" with my address and phone number, and I give them out everywhere. I talk to folks from all over the country. Hopefully we help each other by sharing our experience, our compassion and directions on "where to find out." When I sense I'm helping others I know I'm helping myself more. Statistics prove that support-group members and those who reach out to help others with the same disease live longer and stronger than those who keep to themselves.

Over the past year I have also become heavily involved in the local Wellness Community, a national organization with roots in California (Gilda Radner made it famous). All cancer survivors are welcome. All services are free of charge. The Wellness Community offers therapy groups, yoga, meditation and relaxation classes, children's groups, caretakers' therapy groups, nutrition seminars, couples sharing groups, men's groups, breast-cancer groups, and more. My involvement with the Wellness Community has become one of the most important components of helping to achieve my state of mind, my contentment with my life. I highly recommend participation.

It is coming up to nine years since my original diagnosis. I have learned a lot about prostate cancer, about me, about my purpose in life, about appreciating my miracles — my wife, children and grandchildren. I have learned to advocate for myself and to help others. My life is no longer one long job, trying to earn more and more money. I am grateful for the life I live today. Having cancer for me has a positive side. My fondest desire is to assist others to find the peace, pride and fulfillment I have found.

Harry B. Harris

Retired U.S. Army lieutenant colonel
Silver Spring, Md.

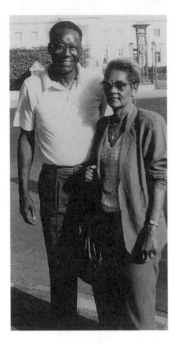

Harry Harris and his wife, Anna.

Diagnosed with prostate cancer at age 69

As a retired U.S. Army lieutenant colonel, it was my custom to get a haircut every 10 to 14 days. It was a delightful October day in 1991 when I drove to the barber shop, located on the campus of the Walter Reed Army Medical Center. As I walked into the lobby, I glanced at the newspaper rack and saw the publication *Stripe*, published in the interest of the patients and staff of Walter Reed. Being an avid reader, I picked up a copy and continued toward the barber shop. As I flipped through, I noticed an article entitled "Prostate Examinations Prove Lifesaving." Initially, I felt that the article did not apply to me, but I decided to read it while waiting for my haircut. I had never been sick one day in my life, felt good and had kept up a daily routine of exercise after military retirement.

The statement "early detection is the key to successful treatment" stuck with me as I continued to read the article, even though I still felt that my health condition was anything but cancerous, because I had lived what I thought was a very good life. I had never smoked, was a teetotaler (still am), had always had a sound diet and had not suffered any environmental risk, other than World War II, Korea, Vietnam, and various overseas assignments during my 20 years as a U.S. Foreign Service officer.

But my optimism descended to earthly realism when I read about the possible warning signs of prostate cancer, which included:

• difficulty or inability to urinate;
• frequent urination, especially at night;

- pain or burning upon urination or ejaculation; and
- the presence of blood or pus in the urine or semen.

I felt a clang of thunder hit me squarely in the face and a bolt of lightning shoot through my spine, and suddenly my whole body became numb as I realized I had experienced all of these symptoms at one time or another. I attributed them to age, or drinking too much water or pop late at night. The one exception was when I passed blood one morning. I was really scared and told my wife about it. She urged me to go to the hospital right away, and I did. The doctor in the general outpatient clinic assured me that it was probably not serious and that I should return for further checkups if it occurred again.

Within a few days of reading that article in *Stripe*, I made an appointment with a urologist, who gave me a digital-rectal examination and a PSA blood test. My PSA was a 7.5, and a subsequent biopsy revealed that I had prostate cancer. I decided on surgery.

I felt no pain and recovered rapidly. I was released from the hospital after several days. I thought that I had taken adequate time for recovery, but I had a minor setback: inability to urinate after the catheter was removed. This indicated that I might have been too hasty in performing certain physical activities after surgery, such as going up the stairs or lifting something that was too heavy. However, after eight months, I was able to carry on a normal life with only minor side effects.

Today my lifestyle remains basically what it was before surgery. My last PSA was less than .01 ng/ml. When weather permits, I continue my daily exercise (walking, jogging) and play golf at least three times a week.

Life can be good after prostate surgery — if there is the desire.

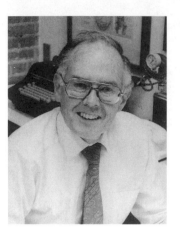

Gerald P. Hodge
Retired art professor
Ann Arbor, Mich.

Diagnosed with prostate cancer at age 74

I often wondered what my thoughts and attitude would be if I were told I had cancer. I assumed that psychologically I would need to have the cancer removed surgically as quickly as possible rather than opt for an alternate treatment. However, when a biopsy of my prostate gland revealed I did have cancer, I discussed the various options with my doctor and settled for cryosurgery.

Never one to put off worrisome things, I was able to have the procedure done within a few days — on Christmas Eve — rather than wait until after the holidays.

It was necessary to be in the hospital for only one night. The two inconveniences were having a small catheter placed through my lower abdomen into my bladder for about 10 days and having my scrotal area very swollen, as was expected. This was inconvenient because sitting was somewhat painful and I spent much of the first couple of weeks in bed. I even devised a donut-shaped pillow so I could sit up and eat. I have never had major surgery, but I think the trauma and period of recovery from cryosurgery would be about the equivalent of abdominal surgery.

In time, with the prostate gland somewhat shrunken, I no longer had the need to urinate frequently at night. Before cryosurgery, I had to get up from four to five times a night. Now, I only need to urinate once or twice a night, so I am very pleased.

In about six months, my PSA reading climbed a few points and a biopsy showed there were a few new cancer cells in my prostate gland. In discussing the various choices for treatment again, this time radiation seemed to suit me best. The treatment was convenient, easy, pleasant, and I looked forward to chatting with the same patients during my seven weeks of treatment. Being a private person, I did not inform any of my friends or relatives of my condition or treatment, and I became quite adept at making excuses if something else came up at the time of treatment — although the people in the radiation oncology department were very nice about changing my schedule if I had another important appointment.

Because of the position of my cancer, some of the rays also focused on my lower rectal area, and about two-thirds of the way through my treatment, I had pain and some bleeding with each bowel movement. The pain subsided after several months, although a small amount of bleeding persists after seven months. Otherwise there have been no side effects from the radiation. My PSA reading three months after radiation therapy was 2.3, and after seven months it decreased to 1.1.

I am rather surprised that during my two types of treatment, my overall attitude was always positive and my worries were minimal. In part, I attribute this to the caring attitudes of the doctors and technicians, and the feeling that I was receiving the best treatment available. I feel that radiation therapy was a good choice for my second go-around, and perhaps cryosurgery was also instrumental in my cure. For both procedures I experienced no bladder incontinence. Healthwise, I feel wonderful and have no complaints.

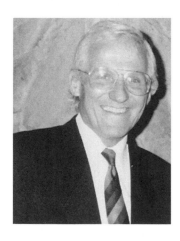

Richard J. Howe, Ph.D.

Engineer
Houston, Texas

Diagnosed with prostate cancer at age 62

My case is a relatively simple one. My first and only PSA test, at age 62, was a 4.2. My urologist performed a transrectal ultrasound, which was normal. He then performed six needle biopsies, two of which were positive in the left lobe of the gland. The disease was stage B1. After surgery, in mid-1991, the disease was upstaged to B2 because I was found to have cancer in both lobes, or sides, of the prostate. Currently, my PSA level is stable at less than 0.1.

My doctor allowed me to examine sections of my tumor under a microscope. Two slides showed invasion into but not through the wall of the prostate.

Based on all these findings, I have concluded that I probably had a very close call. No one knows just when the cancer would have penetrated the wall and then spread beyond the tissue removed by the surgeon, but I am apparently not going to have to find out.

What really concerns me as a patient is that at the time of detection, I could have been considered by some to be a candidate for watchful waiting, or expectant management. This would have probably been a serious mistake. When you are looking at your own cancer on your slides, the whole debate about watchful waiting comes into much sharper focus.

As far as side effects from the surgery are concerned, I was left with mild urinary incontinence (stress incontinence) and was left essentially impotent. The incontinence was corrected by a series of six collagen injections. My problem with impotence was originally overcome through the injection of a mixture of vasoactive drugs (papavarine, phentolamine and prostaglandin E1) prior to intercourse. However, these injections became more painful and the pain lasted for longer periods. Therefore, I decided to have a three-piece penile implant last year. This solved the problem and it has continued to operate satisfactorily.

In summary, I am satisfied with my decision to undergo radical surgery and am more than willing to live with the side effects in return for an apparent cure.

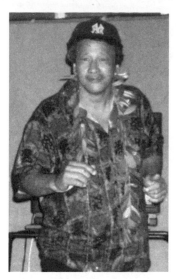

Earl Leslie
Retired drywaller
Kona, Hawaii

Diagnosed with prostate cancer at age 49

One day I noticed blood in my semen and urine. I was a little worried about it, so three days later I went to my regular doctor for a checkup. I found out there was something hard on my prostate, so my doctor referred me to a urologist, who found an infection on my prostate. While being treated for the infection, a blood test revealed that my PSA was high. I had never heard about PSA, but it didn't take me long to find out what it was.

Worry started to move in as I thought about my loved ones: my wife and three beautiful children.

I was told to take a bone scan, and two days later the results came back. Cancer. It had already spread to parts of my bones. Symptoms appeared. My doctor recommended monthly shots or removing my testicles. I chose the shots. Since that day my whole life completely changed. I could no longer do the things that I liked, like diving and fishing. I also had a hard time finding a job. I started to isolate myself from my friends.

I started my treatment, a monthly shot and a pill that shuts off the fuel that feeds the cancer. I also started wearing a pain patch.

By this time I was suffering from insomnia caused by too much stress. I stayed up for about five nights and felt completely drained. Also I suffered from constipation caused by the treatment and pain medication. I went to see an internist who treated me for insomnia. Finally I got my sleep back.

I've started reading books about prostate cancer to learn how I can help myself. I get scared when I read too much about it, especially when I get to the negative parts. I've also started to reach for alternative treatments, such as flaxseed oil and a good, nutritious diet. I'm also reaching out to the Lord for healing. I believe He can do it. I attend church every Sunday and go to a Bible class once a week. My biggest support comes from my pastor, Richard, his wife, Marsa, and my wife and children.

I try to handle my life a day at a time. I'm always hoping and praying for better treatments to come by, if not for now, hopefully sometime soon for future patients. I try to have a good relationship with my doctor.

I used to do a lot of drinking. I don't do it anymore. I learned that it wasn't good for my immune system. I drank for about 25 years. I don't miss it; I feel that my life comes first. I wish I had thought about it long time ago.

I think one of my biggest disappointments since my battle with prostate cancer began has been financial, since I had to stop working. It has taken a lot out of my wife and children, especially my boy who is attending his last year in college. He's had to work 40 hours a week and go to school.

I try to convince family members, friends and even strangers that a prostate checkup is the best hope for survival, and not to take life for granted.

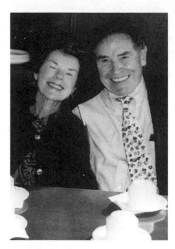

Terry Roe and his wife, Mickey.

Terry Roe

Retired merchandising consultant, Martinsville, N.J.

Diagnosed with prostate cancer at age 65

I am nearly 71 years old and have been a prostate-cancer survivor for five and a half years.

Although the disease struck me in 1991, my ability to deal with it emotionally was aided by events that happened seven years before.

In 1984 while I was working as a consultant in Milan, Italy, I was struck by a severe, life-threatening heart attack. But, while seemingly recovering, I fell into a major depression. I was hospitalized for six weeks in the United States, underwent electroconvulsive therapy and recovered.

The support and love of my wife, Mickey, and our five children was the most positive medicine of all.

When in 1991 I was diagnosed with prostate cancer, I was stunned, as if struck by a truck. But, after two days of brooding, I came to grips with myself and the disease. I knew from my past experience that worrying and self-pity didn't work.

I subsequently decided on a radical prostatectomy but this procedure was aborted because the cancer was found to have metastasized to my lymph nodes. Shortly thereafter, radiation therapy was employed for seven weeks, after which I was placed on hormonal therapy.

Once again, the best cure was the nonchalant affection of my wife and family — by now increased to five in-laws and nine grandchildren.

I then joined an US TOO prostate-cancer support group at Memorial Sloan-Kettering Cancer Center in New York and soon found that self-help could be augmented with group support. It was a chance to meet other men afflicted by prostate cancer. I came to realize that, as sorry as I felt for myself, there were other people there with more significant problems than mine.

I sat next to survivors 40 or 50 years old with young families, others with more severe disease. Some men were depressed and others could count their mortality in months — not years.

Other well-adjusted survivors pepped me up and I was transformed from a receiver of help to a giver. I became an activist in the prostate-cancer-support movement, serving as a regional director of US TOO and the Prostate Cancer Support Network. My mission is to help start support groups in the New York/New Jersey area. Practically every day I receive a phone call from a newly diagnosed man and we share, in a personal way, our common ailment. We chat about something that is new and strange to them but a constant companion to me.

Women get prostate cancer too! They suffer the same terrifying emotions as their spouse — perhaps more so. How often I've chaired support-group meetings and have heard men complain of sexual dysfunction while next to each of them sits their wife — silent — who suffers from the same rupture in a loving physical relationship. Sons in the same family may suddenly find themselves at future risk because of a genetic predisposition to the disease. Is it any wonder that survivors refer to prostate cancer as a family disease?

Education about the disease is sorely needed by many undiagnosed Americans, but to those men and survivors it must be made clear that from an emotional point of view, prostate cancer can be dealt with.

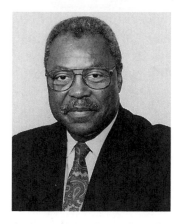

Robert J. Samuels

Retired banker and founder, Tampa Bay Men's Cancer Task Force. President, National Prostate Cancer Coalition Tampa, Fla.

Diagnosed with prostate cancer at age 56

In September 1994, I was working as a small-business consultant for the Greater Tampa Chamber of Commerce. One day while having lunch with one of my colleagues at the chamber, he informed that he had just been diagnosed with prostate cancer. This was the first time I had ever spoken to someone who admitted they had been diagnosed with cancer. I began to ask him questions: How can you tell you have cancer? What are some of the physical symptoms? How do you treat this cancer? How much time do you have left? That lunch conversation motivated me to contact my general practitioner and request a physical examination.

About a week later, I visited my physician. He took some blood samples and suggested I call back in a week for the results. I called the following week and was informed that my PSA level was elevated, and he suggested I consult with a urologist. Prior to this examination I had never thought I had any reason to visit a urologist.

A week later, in early October 1994, I contacted a urologist friend of mine and set up an appointment. Upon visiting his office I gave him copies of my medical records, including the results of my PSA test. I still was not sure exactly what PSA meant. My urologist friend proceeded to order a series of tests and suggested we do a biopsy. He explained the procedure would involve using a thin needle to remove small samples from the prostate for examination under a microscope. The following week he performed the biopsy in his office. The probe didn't hurt particularly (I had heard that it was very painful); a lot of the discomfort is psychological rather than physical. Later I learned that many men suffer considerable anxiety over these tests, whether it be from the invasion or the associated discomfort. The following week I was informed that my biopsy came back negative. However, the urologist suggested that because of my high PSA level, I should allow him to do another biopsy, just to double check. This time he would perform the biopsy in the hospital and send the sample upstairs to the hospital lab. A week later I had the second biopsy and within 20 minutes, while still lying on the table, the results came back positive. The doctor then informed me that I had prostate cancer. I wasn't sure what he said after he told me; my initial reaction was shock, confusion, fear, anger, depression, self-pity — how could this happen to me? The only question I could think to ask the doctor at that time was: How much time do I have left? To me cancer was synonymous with death.

Bankers take great pride in their ability to listen, analyze information and make what they think are well-thought-out, godlike decisions. Bankers speak a language that most laymen would find difficult to fully understand. We can speak for hours about economic indicators, joint ventures, leverage buyouts, cogeneric mergers, conversion ratios, accelerated depreciation, coefficient of variation, correlation coannuities, reverse repos and all types of financial mumbo jumbo. But when it came to prostate cancer, I was just another untutored, under-read, medically ignorant patient, half traumatized from the shocking news of his prostate cancer. How was I supposed to help participate in my own treatment choices? I barely knew a prostate from a kidney and couldn't tell an aspirin from a Tylenol. How was I to choose a treatment?

But I did understand two of the terms my doctor used: cancer and impotence. The first week after I was diagnosed is still vivid in my mind. It was the longest, hardest and loneliest week I had to endure in my struggle with prostate cancer. In addition to personally coming to grips with this disease and my own emotional reaction to it, how was I to break the news to the people who were closest to me, primarily my three sons, my mom and dad and, most of all, the woman I love? I realized that this disease would not only affect me, but all the people who love and care about me.

While discussing my situation with some of my friends, I discovered that quite a few men I knew had been treated for prostate cancer. Some of these men were close friends, and I was stunned to learn that they had been treated but had never mentioned anything about their disease. I told my friends that had I known about their prostate-cancer experience, I would have been more aware of the risks of prostate cancer. I decided right then that the conspiracy of silence and hiding in the closet was going to stop with me. At this point I made up my mind to develop a men's cancer task force and speak out publicly about this disease. As a result of that meeting we created the Tampa Bay Men's Cancer Task Force.

All serious illness disrupts one's life and is accompanied by a variety of emotions, including anger, confusion, depression and loss of control. Among these, the one constant is uncertainty, which brings fear — fear of the impact on relationships with friends and family, fear of treatment and its side effects, fear of how one's life might be changed forever and, ultimately, fear of pain and death. It is the unknown and the uncertain future that makes a serious illness so frightening. All of these feelings are normal and are experienced to greater or lesser degrees by patients with cancer.

Knowledge of your disease and having a positive attitude toward your treatment may help you control some of your emotional and physical reaction to it. Some studies have shown that learning more about your illness and treatment options helps you take a more active part in your care.

The most important thing that you, as a patient or family member, can do when making a treatment decision is to know the facts about your disease. Understand that you have choices and you must be up to date on the latest information available to help you make the best choice. Don't feel guilty for questioning your physician's advice, and ask that all options be fully explained to you.

It is important that you take an active part in your treatment by asking questions and expressing your feelings. Your most valuable tool in coping with cancer is your knowledge and understanding of the disease.

C

Is prostate cancer
a worldwide epidemic?

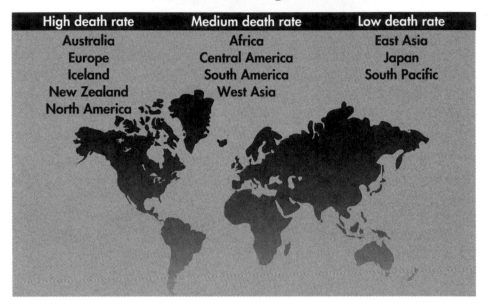

High death rate	Medium death rate	Low death rate
Australia	Africa	East Asia
Europe	Central America	Japan
Iceland	South America	South Pacific
New Zealand	West Asia	
North America		

Fig. 11C — Prostate Cancer: a Global View

The worldwide distribution of death rates for prostate cancer.

The world's population is getting older, which means that some of the trends in prostate cancer seen in the United States are already taking hold around the world. Europe will lose nearly 100,000 men to prostate cancer in the year 2000. Men diagnosed today in China have a much more aggressive disease and have a greater chance of dying from it compared to a man diagnosed in this country. In Russia, the majority of men diagnosed with prostate cancer have advanced disease. Hundreds of thousands of men will have died of prostate cancer around the world by the year 2000. Indeed, prostate cancer is a worldwide epidemic (see Fig. 11C).

Men around the world feel the same stresses as men in the United States who are affected by the disease. A study out of Stockholm, Sweden measured cortisol levels (a steroid that reflects the level of stress a person is feeling) in men going through prostate-cancer screening. Of 2,400 men evaluated, it was found that those undergoing screening had higher quantities of cortisol in their blood than those who were not being screened for prostate cancer. The mere suggestion of such a test appeared to increase their stress. Even higher cortisol levels were found in men waiting on biopsy results. In both the screened and biopsied men, cortisol levels decreased after they were given their results.

The stories you are about to read come from men around the world. They represent a variety of ages and treatments. They are just a few of the millions worldwide who have been diagnosed with prostate cancer in the past decade.

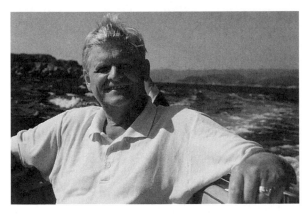

Gunnar Fonne
Research chemist
Oslo, Norway

Diagnosed with advanced prostate cancer at age 60

Prologue
In 1990, a small company I owned had to be sold and eventually I went bankrupt. It never occurred to me that finding a new job would be difficult. I soon discovered that not only was I unattractive professionally because of my age, but Norway was in a deepening depression and there simply weren't any jobs to be had.

The following years were very difficult financially, although we always managed to make ends meet, as my wife worked as a secretary while pursing a college degree. Eventually we decided to emigrate to Canada, as my wife's family lives in Montréal. We lived with them while I looked for work. I found a job, but soon after the company folded. Back to square one. In 1992 I was recruited for a very prestigious and well-paying job in Oslo, so naturally I jumped at the chance and returned home. This job lasted for a little under two years. Fortunately, my contract tided me over until I found the job I have now as a consultant for a research institute. Meanwhile, my mother died at the age of 89 after a gradual and painful decline of her faculties.

It was the following year, in November of 1994, that I found out I had prostate cancer.

I have given such a detailed account of my job problems because I have come to believe that to a large extent the constant struggles and disappointments I have been through have played a major part in the development of my disease.

I have a strong sense of duty. My upbringing has taught me the importance of providing for my family and fulfilling my responsibilities to them as well as to my employer. For years I felt I had to bear all setbacks and disappointments with a stiff upper lip. Everyone thought I was an incurable optimist.

The diagnosis

I had not been feeling well for some time. Because of excruciating pains in my back, I went to see a urologist. When I heard the diagnosis, I was somehow expecting it. My immediate reaction was that I was ready. My family was provided for, the children almost finished with their degrees and well on their way in life. As a matter of fact, I felt sort of relaxed. My scientific brain rationalized it to be a very natural and statistically correct time for my life to end.

The doctor advised me to take it easy and wait and see. The monthly injections seemed noninvasive. I could even continue working without anyone being the wiser. My wife was with me when I received the diagnosis but I didn't want anyone else to know. After a great deal of pleading, she convinced me to tell the children at least, but no one else was told, not even my sisters.

After the diagnosis

The first year went pretty smoothly, but then slowly the pains started coming back. I had more radiation treatment in February 1996 on my lower back, but by April I was back in the hospital and was put on pain killers while they tested me in every possible way to find the immediate cause of the pain. The tests showed no change. I was finally released without receiving any further treatment. But by now I was on constant pain medication. A trip to the South, in the hopes of finding a little relief, was a disaster. My nerves were raw at this point and I started getting bouts of depression, which I've never had, despite my past financial difficulties. Lots of repressed feelings surfaced — regrets and disappointments. On our return from vacation my legs gave way. I was rushed to the hospital and the MRI showed metastascs in my spine.

At this point, something radical seemed to be happening inside me. Suddenly all my relationships seemed to take on a new meaning. It dawned on me that my role as a partner and source of comfort and love was far from over. I felt I had so much more to give my family and I realized that they still needed me. It was like a new world had opened up in front of me.

But how could I have missed all the signals that must have been bombarding me all along? I must have been blind. Or perhaps I allowed my goals to overshadow everything. I had thought I was being rational and down to earth, as a scientist with my background and upbringing should be. I prided myself on being the problem-solver in the family, so I wanted to handle things my way and felt that I knew best.

But I was wrong on many counts. I certainly realize now, at last, that a new struggle has started. The fight is on again. My illness has helped me focus on getting back to my life again, back to my family and friends. I know I need all the support I can get — and am getting — from my family and friends, and hopefully from the medical profession.

It has been a great help to me to put my thoughts down on paper. It's rather like writing the minutes of a meeting; it allows me to close one chapter before looking forward to the next.

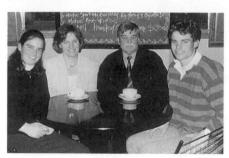

Peter Hart (third from left) with his family.

Peter L. Hart

School teacher
Frankston, Victoria, Australia

Diagnosed with advanced prostate cancer at age 55

I suppose the biggest effect that has been brought about by having prostate cancer is the change in the relationship between my wife, Pam, and me. The closeness of our relationship has varied, and we have had to work hard to try and understand each other again. The medication I am taking to treat this cancer (Zoladex and flutamide) has seemed to take away my sexual desires. We need to be able to express our needs and desires physically, and this has often been hard to do.

As each day goes by I try to address the problem. I don't ever seem to be able to put the cancer out of my mind. I do seem to have good days and bad days. Whether this is the cancer or the medication I use, I am not sure.

I know at the moment I feel quite well. I know I have the support of my family as well as many friends who constantly ask how I am. I also know that I have excellent doctors I can turn to. There is no doubt that attitude is important, and every time a "hiccup" comes along we say, "We're going to fight this together."

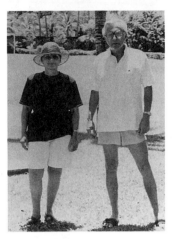

Dr. Clodomiro Mora and his wife, Myrna.

Dr. Clodomiro Mora

Periodontist
San Jose, Costa Rica

Diagnosed with prostate cancer at age 66

As of this writing in 1996, I am in the process of deciding which treatment to ask for. Before deciding which course to take, I am learning all I can on the subject so that I don't feel badly toward myself or my urologist over the final outcome of my chosen treatment or its secondary effects.

There is very little information available to the public about the prostate; on the contrary, contradictions and false information are widespread. There are discrepancies about what to do and how to handle the situation.

During this stressful period I have sometimes slept badly and have had frequent nightmares. My family worries and suffers.

Much has been accomplished with regard to the early detection of prostate tumors, but this progress has not been accompanied by a precise method of determining prognosis and procedures for treatment.

Increasing public awareness about prostatic disease is a primary need. The subject of prostate cancer makes many people feel uncomfortable, so they may avoid discussing it altogether.

It has not been easy to find people willing to talk about the subject. It would be a great help and serve as an important source of information if groups could be formed in Costa Rica by those who have had prostate problems or are currently experiencing them.

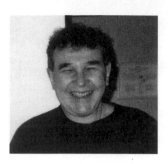

Norm Oman
Retired school teacher
Winnipeg, Manitoba, Canada

Diagnosed with advanced prostate cancer at age 62

I discovered a lump on a testicle at 7:36 a.m. Dec. 17, 1992. (Some dates just stick in the mind.) Any lump on the body is a concern, but on a testicle!

My general practitioner looked, felt, and referred me to a urologist. The urologist looked, felt, poked and took blood. He also booked an ultrasound. Back in the urologist's office, I got the results. The lump was inconsequential — a hydrocele (whatever the hell that was). However, the blood test showed a PSA of 25.

"A what of what? What's a PSA? What does 25 mean?"

What it meant was I was scheduled for a biopsy, another ultrasound and another blood test.

Ultrasound: O.K.

PSA: 24.

Biopsy: one core positive.

Gleason: 5.

The urologist said "CANCER." I went deaf and asked for a second opinion. Dr. Second Opinion confirmed Dr. First Opinion and told me the options — radical prostatectomy or radiation. Dr. First Opinion said some nonsense about castration. Dr. First Opinion told me not to worry about anything.

Off to surgery. Surgery aborted; lymph nodes cancerous. New ball game — but I get to keep my prostate. Start on CHT (combined hormone therapy). Zoladex and flutamide. The flutamide caused serious diarrhea, so they put me on Androdur.

By the way — shortly after leaving the hospital my left leg swelled up and became quite painful. Diagnosis: lymphocele. Lucky me.

Where am I today? My lymphocele has been successfully treated. I've been off active cancer treatment (hormonal) for 15 months, but my PSA has risen from 0.25 to 6.25.

I cycle, play squash, exercise and visit with my grandchildren. I'm nervous and frightened by my cancer. I wish there were more effective treatments after hitting the wall with hormone therapy. Isn't that where research should be more focused?

What helps me now? My wife. The prostate-cancer support group I'm involved with. Working with the support group movement — and just trying.

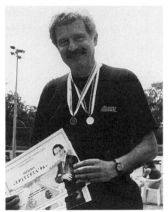

George Nicholas Stathopoulos

Private international lawyer
Athens, Greece

Diagnosed with prostate cancer at age 57

I was diagnosed with prostate cancer four years ago by pure chance when I went to a family doctor for a general physical. Among other tests, he suggested the PSA blood test, as warranted by my age.

It was then, in April 1991, that I first heard of PSA. Before that, neither I nor any of my friends had heard of it.

My first PSA reading was 6.5. When I saw the results, I got worried. I immediately went to a urologist, who gave me a rectal examination and said I shouldn't worry; it was probably an inflammation. I got another reading a month later and it was 7.5. Although the doctors still said it was probably nothing to worry about, I was not satisfied. I started reading everything I could find about prostate cancer. There was a lot there!

After another two PSA tests a month apart, 6.5 and 10, respectively, I was advised to undergo an ultrasound and biopsy.

Soon after, while on holiday on the Greek island of Kea, I received the bad news. A secretary in my office had received a fax from my urologist, and she in turn faxed it to me. When the fax started to come through, you can imagine my anxiety. When I saw more than one page, I knew I had cancer even before reading the results. I was shocked and shaking and said to my wife that I needed a drink to calm me down. But soon my mind moved on to action, and a month later, in mid-September 1991, I was referred to the Mayo Clinic.

After weighing the pros and cons of surgery and radiation, my wife and I decided on total prostatectomy, since I was only 57 years old, athletic and in otherwise excellent health. It was then and is very clear to me today that this was the best way to go in my case.

Soon after my recovery, which was quick, I started telling all of my friends all over the world to have the PSA test. I felt that I was lucky that by mere chance my prostate cancer had been confined in the gland and that it could be removed.

Not long after my operation I started participating in sports again, including jogging, tennis and basketball, something I had never stopped since my University of Michigan track days with my then track coach and now good friend Don Canham.

A couple of years ago, I started training for the Senior Pan European Championship here in Athens. Due to a knee injury, I didn't compete, but on the advice of another senior track participant, I started competing in the shot put and discus at various Greek national meets. Last year at the outdoor National Greek Championships I won the shot put and came in third in the discus. This year, I won gold and silver medals in both events.

I suppose, in a way, I wanted to prove to myself that I had conquered cancer and would not let anything interfere with my normal life as an international lawyer and as a family man with my American wife, Margaret, and three beautiful bicultural children, Angeliki-Anna, Katerina and Nicholas.

I believe I have achieved this. I continue to work on Greek and European community issues, to take part in seminars and handle delicate issues with the same energy I had before the cancer.

I continue to tell everyone I know about the importance of the PSA test and rectal exam. Both are necessary. If there is evidence of cancer from either test, one should go for a biopsy and not waste time waiting for something to happen. It's best to know as soon as possible, before prostate cancer spreads.

I also advise patients and families that if there is cancer, everyone in the family should know. You can't hide it and there is no shame. It can happen to anyone.

When everyone is informed, the whole process becomes easier. When I was diagnosed, we told the children about it and assured them it was caught early enough and was curable. Even our then 4-year-old son, Nicholas, had a good idea of what it was all about.

I feel that going through a cancer experience and having it behind you somehow gives you more strength in all aspects of life. It also makes you more philosophical. In my case, I feel that small things aren't worth worrying about, as there is so much beauty in life itself and I feel very grateful to be as I am today, in excellent physical and mental health.

Prostate cancer hasn't slowed me down in any way. In fact, it may have given me a second wind to enjoy life, family, friends, and interests such as art, music and travel.

Finally, my advice is that if you get the bad news, stay calm, find out all you can about the illness, consult a good physician, decide on which way to go, and do it — with courage.

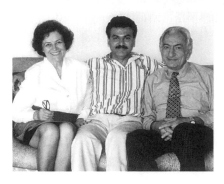

Ghanin Toma

Retired businessman
Barcelona, Spain

Diagnosed with prostate cancer
at age 64

Ghanin Toma (far right)
with his wife, Magda, and
nephew, Namir Stephan.

For years, my annual prostate checkups consisted of only a digital-rectal exam, or DRE. And in December 1993 I was reading a *Time* magazine article on PSA testing and so I decided to go back to my doctor and ask for a DRE *and* a PSA. My DRE was normal but my PSA was 5.6. I decided to get a second opinion three months later. Again, the DRE was negative but my PSA was now 5.8. An ultrasound was also done but this turned out to be negative.

I did not want to think much about it, but I became preoccupied. I had a feeling that something was wrong even though many of the tests showed that things were OK.

In December 1994, I went to see another doctor. Another ultrasound and DRE turned out to be negative, but my PSA was now 6.5. I decided to see more doctors, have more tests and get even more opinions.

Finally, in June 1995, my PSA became 7.8 (with a negative DRE and ultrasound, of course) and so my wife and I insisted to the doctor that a biopsy be done. The biopsy indicated cancer (Gleason score of 5).

That little feeling I had in the back of my mind had been right. I was worried but I decided to really go out and find the best treatment, and when all was said and done here was my scorecard: The number of doctors I visited before the biopsy? Five. The number of doctors I visited after diagnosis for possible treatment advice? Eight.

Most of the doctors that I talked to wanted me to have surgery or radiation (depending, of course, on who I talked to, a urologist or a radiologist). So, I read some more articles, considered my age, and the fact that all of the doctors agreed that I had a life expectancy of at least 15 to 20 more years. In the end I decided to have a radical prostatectomy.

A few days after surgery I went home and, except for a little incontinence, today I am doing fine. I was also lucky to have found a surgeon that does this type of operation all the time, which could have reduced the chances of other side effects.

My wife has been my strength. At first when I was diagnosed I thought I could go through this alone. I did not want her to worry. However, after all is said and done, I cannot imagine having gone through this without her. She slept in a small chair for three nights when I was in the hospital recovering from my surgery! She always goes to her doctor for an annual breast exam and so it motivates me even more to go and see my physician. I have been married for 33 years and because I feel that I have been cured, I am confident that we will celebrate many, many more anniversaries and happy moments.

I advise all men diagnosed with this disease to seek several opinions about treatment and to read as many books about prostate cancer as possible. You have to take control of this disease and learn as much as you can.

Ever since I was diagnosed I have encouraged many neighbors and family members to go and get a prostate checkup. So, I guess the one good thing about being diagnosed with prostate cancer is that if you are very vocal about your disease it may later save someone's life.

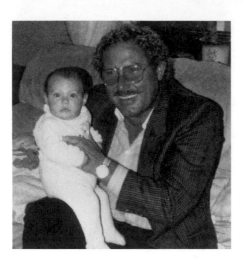

Fred Wedell with his niece Naira.

Fred Wedell

*Director of a biological products company
Dresden, Germany*

Diagnosed with prostate cancer at age 61

My name is Fred Wedell. I am 62 years old and in the best of health, but I used to have prostate cancer.

My tumor was detected by chance during a routine physical. I had an elevated PSA and therefore consulted a urologist for a detailed examination. The urologist could not find any signs of an alteration of the prostate on the ultrasound. I had no symptoms of urinary obstruction and therefore he assumed prostatitis rather than a tumor.

The urologist did a biopsy in order to be sure, and the result shocked me because a prostate cancer was diagnosed. At the urgent advice of my doctor I contacted the university hospital in my hometown to schedule a radical prostatectomy. There I had the opportunity to talk with the assistant medical director about the operation. He explained the operation technique they would use. He also told me that the radical prostatectomy would consequently result in impotence. This statement frightened me and I asked him if it would be possible to bypass the impotence. We had following dialogue:

Doctor: How old are you?

Me: 61 years.

Doctor: What do you want at 61? Do you want potency or cure?

Me: If possible, both.

Then I asked about his age.

Doctor: 39 years.

Me: Sir, that is the age I feel like.

Doctor: With this operation technique it is impossible to prevent impotence.

The next days I was very demoralized about the possibility of becoming cured by surgery on the one hand but losing a very important part of my life on the other. My quality of life would be very restricted.

With a stroke of luck I talked with a friend, a doctor, about my situation. She urged me to contact a urologist she knew in Dresden. During a long discussion I lost my fear. The doctor explained his operation technique and he told me that it could be possible to spare the left nerve so that my potency could be saved — if there were no metastases. After this discussion I had, for the first time, the feeling that everything would be all right.

A biopsy showed that the prostate cancer had the dimension of a pea and that it was indeed confined to the lower right side of the prostate. I had the surgery on March 19, 1996. Thirteen days after surgery the bladder catheter was removed and I could leave the clinic. I had no incontinence. Today, three months after surgery, I feel fantastic. I am very pleased that my potency is getting better and I hope that I can resume a normal sex life.

Today I know how important it is to have a positive attitude about the cancer — and the right physician.

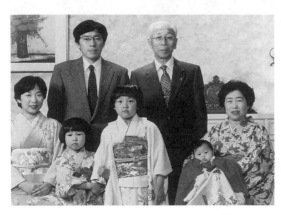

Seiji Yoshimura, M.D., (standing, third from left) and his family.

Seiji Yoshimura, M.D.

Radiologist
Bibai, Hokkaido, Japan

Diagnosed with prostate cancer at age 63

At age 63, with two years remaining in active practice as a radiotherapist, I visited the urologist for mild symptoms of prostatism. Everything was normal except my PSA, which was 5 ng/ml. A needle biopsy, which I reluctantly accepted, also turned out to be negative — a big relief for the time being — and I was placed on PSA follow-up. For the next 14 months there was a slow but steady rise in my PSA, from 5.9 to 8.6. A second prostate biopsy showed cancer, with Gleason score of 6.

I could not believe it was happening to me, as I had never smoked, ate a balanced, nutritious diet and drank only in moderation. My condition, early stage prostate cancer, was rather a rarity in Japan.

I searched the medical literature, filled with many divergent opinions about treatment, which left me confused and uncertain. Meanwhile, I was referred to a urologist in the United States, and through an intensive discussion about a broad range of treatments, I decided to have surgery. I was nervous, with ill thoughts about the disease, surgery, outcome and prognosis. My wife and family were nervous as well, but they were also assertive and a big support to me.

Three and a half years ago I underwent radical prostatectomy. My cancer was indeed organ-confined, and it was totally removed.

My latest PSA result was 0.2 ng/ml. My urinary control is perfect. I can enjoy golfing two to three times a week with my wife and friends. Although my erectile function is a little bit on the low side compared to before surgery, I can manage it, and my wife is content. Although several more years are needed before the final outcome of my disease becomes apparent, I feel very confident in its complete cure.

Through this duel with prostate cancer in the past six years I have learned so many things. Of these, the experience of being a cancer patient is the most precious one. I learned so much by being a patient. I must admit to having been a bit ignorant about how patients feel and respond to even the smallest comment by a physician. Although not in full-time practice now, I am a better physician to talk to, and I really listen to each patient.

I am much, much luckier than many other cancer patients, whose terminal course I've witnessed so many times during my practice as a therapeutic radiologist.

As a Buddhist, I pray every morning for the eternal and heavenly peace of those who unfortunately succumbed to death, and I pledge to live to the full extent of my ability and do something positive about the war on cancer, from which I fortunately returned alive.

Medical References

Title: **"Being sensitive to the psychological needs of patients with prostate cancer"**
Authors: Berger, N.S.; and Crawford, E.D.
Journal: *Oncology Nursing Forum*
Volume: 22 (1)
Page: 14
Date: January-February 1995

Title: **"Psychological reactions in men screened for prostate cancer"**
Authors: Gustafsson, O.; Theorell, T.; Norming, U.; et al
Journal: *British Journal of Urology*
Volume: 75
Pages: 631-636
Date: May 1995

Title: **"Quality of life of patients with prostate cancer and their spouses"**
Authors: Kornblith, A.B.; Herr, H.W.; Ofman, U.S.; et al
Journal: *Cancer*
Volume: 73
Pages: 2791-2802
Date: June 1, 1994

Title: **"Men with prostate cancer need psychological support, say patients and physicians"**
Authors: Anonymous
Journal: *Oncology*
Volume: 5 (4)
Page: 39
Date: April 1991

Title: **"Psychological and sexual well-being among prostate cancer patients over time"**
Authors: Cassileth, B.; Soloway, M.; Vogelzang, N.; et al
Journal: *Proceedings from the Annual Meeting: American Society of Clinical Oncology*
Volume: 9
Pages: A-1188
Date: 1990

12

Getting Closer to a Cure

A

What are the latest
advances in diagnosis?

B

What are the newest
methods of staging?

C

What's on the
treatment horizon?

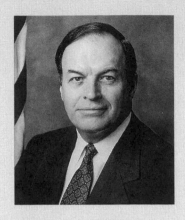

Richard Shelby
U.S. senator

I know how important it is to get screening and early treatment for prostate cancer — I am a prostate-cancer survivor. I had a PSA test, I had a positive score, I had my prostate removed, and I am here to tell about it as a result.

Prostate cancer is a disease that has a similar incidence and death rate to breast cancer yet receives one-fourth as much research money. This is a serious oversight that we should correct to increase the pace of research and develop conclusive evidence on what really works and does not work in treating prostate cancer.

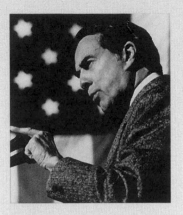

Robert Dole
Former U.S. senator

If I have one message about prostate cancer it is this: There is no doubt that early detection and research save lives. So my advice to every man is to get tested regularly and voice your support of increased funding for prostate cancer research.

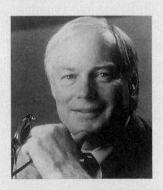

Rep. James A. Leach
U.S. Congress

In my case, timely testing and prompt treatment three years ago has left me problem-free today.

I encourage all people reading this to contact your representatives. A little phone call could make the difference in prostate cancer funding. If we can increase research dollars then I believe we can get that much closer to finding a cure.

A message from the authors

The future of prostate-cancer research and the closer we get to a cure depends neither on medical researchers nor doctors. It depends on you.

Today, the amount of money put aside for research in the United States is directly related to the activity of political special-interest groups. We need to learn from the AIDS and breast-cancer coalitions and look to them as a model and an inspiration. They have worked to unite and request more funding for research — locally, through community fund-raising events; and nationally, through letters or phone calls to their congressional representatives and senators.

Indeed, a single voice can make a dramatic difference. For example, one phone call from a senator in Washington, D.C., in 1996 increased the potential funding of a prostate-cancer research bill from $7 million to $100 million!

Only a few years ago, breast-cancer funding was ridiculously short of what was needed to effectively educate and potentially find a cure. But a group of politically motivated women and men has since assembled to demand more resources, and significant progress has been made. In 1994, for example, the National Institutes of Health funneled $263 million into breast-cancer studies. That same year, the NIH allocated $55 million for research of the prostate gland.

While prostate cancer is still an underdog disease, both politically and scientifically, its researchers can only benefit from the advances being made against other diseases, such as breast cancer and AIDS. That's why research funding in all areas of medicine is crucial, because a discovery in one could have an impact on the understanding of another. For example, the breast-cancer drug Taxol is now being tested as a treatment for prostate cancer.

Although prostate-cancer groups are becoming more unified and are beginning to assemble nationally, we still have a long way to go. That's why individual political involvement is the single greatest contribution that can be made toward realistically finding a cure.

— *Joseph E. Oesterling, M.D. and Mark A. Moyad, M.P.H.*

A

What are the latest advances in diagnosis?

There is plenty of ongoing research to find a better prostate-tumor marker or one that can be used in addition to the PSA test. However, in the years to come there is one test that will be the focus of a lot of attention: the "percent-free" PSA test. It was already mentioned in Chapter 3, Section C, but it definitely merits even more discussion. This test will help to distinguish men with early prostate cancer from those who have an enlarged prostate gland (see Fig. 12A). This test is currently being used experimentally at institutions around the country, and the results are very encouraging. Men who have a PSA value in the so-called "gray zone" (3-10 ng/ml) could have BPH or they could have cancer, and they are good candidates for this new test, which looks at the various types of PSA that are produced by the prostate. In fact, the prostate produces at least six different types of PSA, two of which are found in large quantities in the bloodstream.

As was explained earlier, there is a "free" form of PSA and a "complexed" form. Current tests measure the total amount of free and complexed PSA to give a single PSA value. This newer test measures the quantity of free PSA and compares it to the total amount of PSA, both free and complexed. Research from Scandinavia has shown that measuring the proportion of free to total PSA can give the physician a better idea of whether you have BPH or prostate cancer. Men with BPH have higher amounts of free PSA, whereas men with prostate cancer have higher amounts of the complexed form.

Once the test is widely adopted, future PSA exams will result in two separate scores: one will represent the total PSA level (free plus complexed PSA), which is the current standard; the other will represent the ratio of free to total PSA in the blood (percent-free PSA). Both scores together should significantly improve the diagnosis of prostate cancer.

It is important to keep in mind that with the new percent-free PSA test, the lower your value, the greater your chance of having prostate cancer. This may seem odd, because it is the opposite of the current PSA test, in which higher values are associated with a greater risk of cancer.

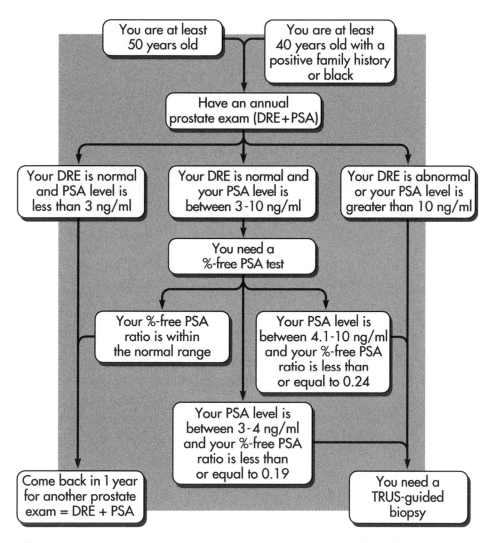

Fig. 12A — The Newest PSA Molecular Forms Flow Chart to Better Determine Whether a Man Has Prostate Cancer

Because the amount of complexed PSA increases with cancer, the ratio of free to total PSA is smaller in men with prostate cancer. For example, if a man without prostate cancer has a free-PSA level of 2 and a total-PSA level of 4, his percent-free PSA ratio would be 0.5 (2/4 = 0.5). On the other hand, if a man with prostate cancer has a free-PSA level of 2 and a total-PSA level of 8, his percent-free PSA ratio would be .25 (2/8 = .25). This lower ratio reflects an increase in complexed PSA, which is a likely indication of prostate cancer.

Because this test is so new, it is impossible to say exactly which institutions offer it, but we do have a list of the companies that are producing the test right now (see Table 12A). This list will undoubtedly grow in the near future.

Table 12A — A List of the Companies That Currently Make the New "Percent-free" PSA Test

Company	Headquarters	Phone number
Abbott Laboratories	Abbott Park, Ill.	(800) 527-1869
Diagnostic Products Corp.	Los Angeles, Calif.	(800) 372-1782
Dianon	Stratford, Conn.	(800) 328-2666
Hybritech Inc.	San Diego, Calif.	(800) 526-3821
Tosoh	Foster City, Calif.	(800) 248-6764
Wallac	Turku, Finland	358-2-2678-111

A new cancer marker called "telomerase" has also been getting a lot of attention. Telomerase is an enzyme that allows cells to grow indefinitely. In theory, the larger the quantity of telomerase detected, the more aggressive the cancer. This finding could then assist in the treatment decision-making process. A recent study from Johns Hopkins demonstrated that 87 percent of prostate-cancer tumors (from biopsy specimens) were positive for telomerase; the enzyme was not detected in normal or BPH tissue. Therefore, telomerase may help in the future detection of prostate cancers, and anti-telomerase therapies one day may be effective.

Finally, a test using a monoclonal antibody to detect the recurrence of prostate cancer is being developed. The monoclonal antibody is a protein that binds only to cancerous prostate tissue. After the antibody is given, an imaging machine similar to that used in a bone scan is used to see whether the antibody has bound to any tissue at or near the surgical site. If such activity is detected, this may be a good indication that the cancer has returned or has spread. A recent study demonstrated that the monoclonal antibody test was six to 10 times more sensitive than CT or MRI scans for detecting prostate-cancer recurrence.

FAST FACT

Currently, more than 100 possible prostate cancer tests are being developed and researched.

B

What are the newest methods of staging?

Some reports indicate that up to 40 percent of patients surgically treated for prostate cancer are clinically "understaged." In other words, the extent and aggressiveness of their cancer was underestimated before surgery. This obviously leaves room for improvement. Therefore, newer staging methods are being used experimentally in many U.S. hospitals.

One such method is called reverse transcriptase-polymerase chain reaction (RT-PCR), or molecular staging. In RT-PCR, a sample of your blood is taken to produce multiple copies of your DNA (deoxyribonucleic acid), or genetic blueprint. The many copies allow the doctor to see if any of the DNA is from prostate-cancer cells that have gained access to your bloodstream. This RT-PCR test is so sensitive that it can detect one prostate-cancer cell hiding amid 100,000 white blood cells. At New York City's Columbia University, research on the effectiveness of this test has been encouraging. Of 65 men who were about to undergo radical prostatectomy, a procedure used exclusively for organ-confined disease, 38 percent were actually found to have cancer that had spread beyond the prostate. Nevertheless, this test is still experimental, and additional research is necessary to determine its true abilities in staging prostate cancer. In the future, this test may be one of the factors that helps to decide whether a patient is a possible candidate for surgery.

Another very promising concept that may be used for staging and possible outcome prediction is the study of angiogenesis, or the ability of a cancer to grow new blood vessels. All cancers have a few things in common; one is that they need a blood supply to keep growing. We now know that cancers can somehow cause blood vessels to grow, and this phenomenon is called angiogenesis ("angio" means "blood vessel" and "genesis" means "to grow"). In fact, we already know that as a prostate cancer moves from one stage to the next, say from a T2b to a T3c, the number of new blood vessels usually increases dramatically (see Fig. 12B). So, future helpful staging

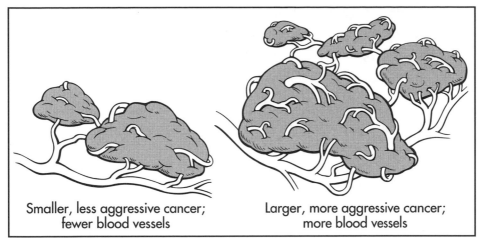

Smaller, less aggressive cancer; fewer blood vessels

Larger, more aggressive cancer; more blood vessels

Fig. 12B — Prostate-cancer Angiogenesis

Analyzing the degree of angiogenesis, or the growth of new blood vessels, is already being tested as a way to stage prostate cancer.

information may be used by just counting the number of vessels within a tumor upon biopsy.

It is theorized that if you can stop the creation of these new blood vessels, then you should be able to stop the growth of the cancer because it is no longer being fed with oxygen-rich blood. Therefore, a large number of antiangiogenesis drugs, or drugs that can potentially stop the growth of new blood vessels, are being tested in many different areas of cancer research, especially prostate cancer (see Table 12B).

Table 12B — Possible Antiangiogenesis Treatments

Category	Example
Anticancer drugs	anti-estrogens, retinoids, interferon, methotrexate, interleukin-12
Anticancer treatments	hyperthermia, radiation therapy
Antibiotics	D-penicillamine, suramin
Others	aspirin, thalidomide, vitamin-D derivatives, angiostatin, endostatin, TNP-470, BB-216, platelet factor 4, carboxyaminotriazole

Two new angiogenesis inhibitors are called "angiostatin" and "endostatin" (discovered at Children's Hospital and Harvard Medical School in Boston, Mass.) Unlike angiogenesis inhibitors of the past, they caused almost total (up to 99 percent) reversal and blockage of cancer growth in mice. In addition, angiostatin did not make the mice sick or produce any drug resistance. These inhibitors can potentially be used during or after chemotherapy and they may also be used for other cancers (such as bladder or breast). Currently, nine different angiogenesis drugs are in phase I or II clinical trials for a host of solid tumors (breast, colon, lung and prostate).

Another predictor of a cancer's aggressiveness is the number of chromosomes within its DNA as compared to the number found in normal human tissue. This calculation, called "ploidy status," is already being used at some institutions to help determine how fast and far prostate cancer may spread.

If the tumor's chromosome count closely resembles that of normal tissue, the cancer is labeled "diploid." Such cancer usually responds very well to treatment such as hormonal therapy. If the cancer's chromosome count is abnormal, the cancer is labeled "aneuploid," which means it has a missing or extra chromosome. Some tumor samples are found to have an extra set of chromosomes, in which case the cancer is called "polyploid." These last two types of cancers tend to be more aggressive and may need more intensive therapy. Limitations of such DNA testing include the possibility of accidentally evaluating noncancerous tissue, which would result in a biopsy being labeled mostly diploid when in reality it could be mostly aneuploid or polyploid.

FAST FACT

Breast cancer is easier to detect on a mammography by the growth of new blood vessels (angiogenesis) in the cancerous tumor.

C
What's on the treatment horizon?

The major problem with hormonal therapy for advanced prostate cancer is that it only works for about three years. After that, the cancer cells develop a resistance to the drugs so they no longer are effective.

One of the most intense areas of medical research surrounds a new way of delivering hormonal therapy that tricks the cancer cells into remaining vulnerable to the drug's effects. The goal is to widen the window of survival for men whose prostate cancer has metastasized, or spread, to other parts of the body.

Called intermittent androgen-deprivation (hormonal) therapy, the treatment involves taking an LHRH agonist and an antiandrogen until your PSA level decreases, and then taking a break from the medication, forcing your body into a so-called "hormonal withdrawal." When your PSA starts to rise again, treatment is resumed. This on-again, off-again drug regimen appears to delay the cancer's ability to start growing again, which may increase the length of survival. Animal studies have proved very promising and early results from human studies should soon be available.

Other treatment possibilities that may help patients with advanced disease include suramin (as mentioned in Chapter 8), which can block certain growth factors that may encourage prostate cancer to grow and spread. So far, however, the research on suramin has been inconclusive. It has been shown to stop some prostate cancers from spreading for a few months and it has been shown to make some patients worse. Suramin also suppresses the immune system, which increases the risk of infections and other complications.

Gene therapy is another hopeful area of prostate-cancer research. There are currently three ways in which gene therapy may help patients with prostate cancer:

- by establishing normal control of cell division, which could be done by inserting genes that suppress tumor development;
- by administering toxic products that target prostate cancer cells; and
- by boosting the immune system. This could be done by inserting tumor genes that the body recognizes as foreign, causing the immune system to kill all cancers related to the gene.

In fact, the greatest promise right now is with a potential vaccine that will soon be tested in men with advanced prostate cancer. In this study, prostate-cancer cells will be removed during routine prostatectomy, genetically modified to trick the immune system into fighting the cancer as if it were a foreign invader, and then be given back to the patient with a simple injection (see Fig. 12C). Studies in rats with advanced prostate cancer have shown a 30-percent long-term cure rate after just three injections.

Researchers at Johns Hopkins University and other institutions recently discovered that chromosome 1 contains the gene for the familial (inherited) form of prostate cancer. Therefore, the actual gene for familial prostate cancer should be discovered very soon.

Genetic changes in chromosomes 8, 10, 16 and 17 also have been associated with prostate cancer, and researchers are attempting to locate the exact genes involved. In addition, recently a metastasis suppressor gene has been found in rat prostate-cancer cells; scientists are trying to find its human equivalent.

The future is prevention

Another promising study, which began in 1993 and will end up being one of the largest clinical trials in U.S. history, is the Prostate Cancer Prevention Trial. In this 10-year study, 18,000 men without prostate cancer are either being given a medication called Proscar (already used for the treatment of BPH; see Chapter 4), which shrinks the prostate and may prevent prostate cancer, or they are taking a placebo. A list of other potential treatments appears in Table 12C.

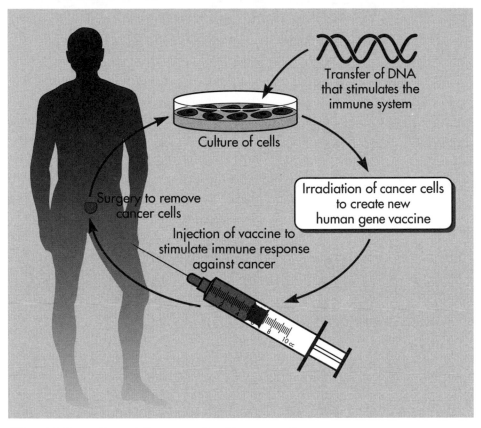

Fig. 12C — Gene Therapy for Prostate Cancer

Clinical trials will soon begin on a gene therapy "vaccine" that stimulates the immune system against prostate cancer in men with advanced disease.

For the latest information on promising treatments and/or upcoming clinical trials for prostate cancer, call your local university-affiliated research institution. Another way to learn about the newest therapies is by contacting national, regional and local support groups.

Table 12C — Future Treatment Possibilities
(For updates call 1-800-4-CANCER)

Drugs Currently Being Tested in Clinical Trials

Aromatase inhibitors (enzymes that convert androgens to estrogens, female hormones)

Cpt-11

Didemnin b

Interferon

Lovastatin (a cholesterol-lowering drug)

Selenium plus vitamin E

Strontium

Suramin

Taxol

Taxotere

Topotecan

Vitamin-A derivatives (retinoids)

Drugs in Development

Timp-2 treatments (may block metastasis)

TGF-beta stimulators (inhibit cancer growth)

Tyrosine kinase blockers (signal other cells)

Treatments Currently Being Tested in Clinical Trials

External-beam radiation therapy

Hormone therapy prior to either prostatectomy or radiation

Hormone therapy vs. observation after radical prostatectomy

Intermittent hormone therapy

Radioactive-seed implants

Radiation vs. observation after prostatectomy

FAST FACT

The National Cancer Institute is planning a study that will evaluate 350,000 individuals to see if what they eat can prevent or slow the growth of prostate, breast or large-bowel cancers.

The ABCs of CHAPTER 12

A Quick Review

A

What are the latest advances in diagnosis?

- The "percent-free" PSA test (also mentioned in Chapter 3, Section C) will help to distinguish men with early prostate cancer from men who have an enlarged prostate gland, or BPH. This test is being used experimentally at institutions around the country.

- The "percent-free" PSA test measures the quantity of free PSA and compares it to the total amount of PSA. If a man has a total PSA level between 3-4 ng/ml and the percent-free PSA level is less than or equal to 0.19, this is abnormal and he needs to have a biopsy. Also, if a man has a total PSA level between 4.1-10 ng/ml and his percent-free PSA is less than or equal to 0.24, this is also abnormal and he needs to have a biopsy.

- A new cancer marker called "telomerase" has also been getting a lot of attention. Telomerase is an enzyme that allows cells to grow indefinitely. In theory, the larger the quantity of telomerase detected, the more aggressive the cancer, which could then help in the treatment decision making process.

B

What are the newest methods of staging?

- The reverse transcriptase-polymerase chain reaction (RT-PCR) test can detect cancerous cells that have gained entry to the blood-stream. In the future, the RT-PCR test could play a major role in determining the best candidates for surgery: those with local-ized disease.

- Angiogenesis is the ability of a cancer to generate new blood vessels so it can receive the nutrients it needs to grow. The greater the number of new blood vessels, the more aggressive the cancer and the more it may spread.

- DNA analysis of the cancer biopsy (DNA ploidy) can determine whether the cancer cells are genetically similar to normal tissue, which means it may not grow quickly; or whether its DNA content is very different, which indicates it may be aggressive.

C

What's on the treatment horizon?

- Intermittent androgen-deprivation therapy is a newer method of treatment for advanced or metastatic prostate cancer. Hormonal therapy is given until the PSA level decreases, and then it is stopped. When the PSA level starts rising again, another dose of hormonal therapy is given, and so on.

- Suramin has shown some promise in treating patients with advanced disease. However, it has also been a disappointment in other studies. Therefore, the overall benefits (if any) of taking this drug are not yet known.

- The best way of participating in a clinical trial or just learning about the most up to date information on the newest treatments is to call your local university-affiliated hospital or a national, regional or local support group. For example, gene-therapy research for prostate cancer has begun recently at several universities and clinical trials for gene therapy should begin very soon.

Medical References

Title: **"Hormone and antihormone withdrawal: implications for the management of androgen-independent prostate cancer"**
Authors: Scher, H.I.; Zhang, Z.F.; Nanus, D.; et al
Journal: *Urology*
Volume: 47 (1A Suppl)
Pages: 61-69
Date: January 1996

Title: **"Free, complexed, and total serum prostate-specific antigen: the establishment of appropriate reference ranges for their concentrations and ratios"**
Authors: Oesterling, J.E.; Jacobsen, S.J.; Klee, G.G.; et al
Journal: *Journal of Urology*
Volume: 154 (3)
Pages: 1090-1095
Date: September 1995

Title: **"Intermittent androgen suppression in the treatment of prostate cancer: a preliminary report"**
Authors: Goldenberg, S.L.; Bruchovsky, N.; Gleave, M.E.; et al
Journal: *Urology*
Volume: 45 (5)
Pages: 839-844
Date: May 1995

Title: **"Molecular staging of prostate cancer with the use of an enhanced reverse transcriptase-PCR assay"**
Authors: Katz, A.E.; Olsson, C.A.; Raffo, A.J.; et al
Journal: *Urology*
Volume: 43 (6)
Pages: 765-775
Date: June 1994

Title: **"Gene therapy for urologic cancer"**
Authors: Sanda, M.; and Simons, J.W.
Journal: *Urology*
Volume: 44 (4)
Pages: 617-624
Date: October 1994

Notes _____

_____

_____

_____

_____

_____

_____

_____

_____

_____

_____

_____

_____

_____

_____

_____

_____

_____

Suggested Reading
and Resources

Books
(Listed by year)

"Going the Distance: One Man's Journey to the End of His Life"
By George Sheehan, M.D.
Random House, New York, N.Y., 1996

"Man to Man: Surviving Prostate Cancer"
By Michael Korda
Random House, New York, N.Y., 1996

"Prostate Cancer"
By American Cancer Society
Random House, New York, N.Y., 1996

"Prostate Disease: The Most Comprehensive, Up-to-Date Information Available to Help You Understand Your Condition, Make the Right Treatment Choices and Cope Effectively"
By William Scott McDougal and P.J. Skerrett
Times Books, New York, N.Y., 1996

"The Patient's Guide to Prostate Cancer"
By Marc B. Garnick Jr.
Plume Publishers, a Division of Penguin Books U.S.A. Inc., 1996

"Me Too: A Doctor Survives Prostate Cancer"
By James E. Payne
WRS Publishing, Waco, Texas, 1995

"Prostate & Cancer: A Family Guide to Diagnosis, Treatment & Survival"
By Sheldon Marks
Fisher Books, Tucson, Ariz., 1995

"Solving Prostate Problems: Answers and Advice From a Leading Expert"
By Martin K. Gelbard and William Bentley
Simon & Schuster, New York, N.Y., 1995

"The Prostate: A Guide for Men and the Women
Who Love Them"
> *By Patrick C. Walsh and Janet Farrar Worthington*
> *The Johns Hopkins University Press, Baltimore, Md., 1995*

"Choices" (Pages 376-405)
> *By Marion Morra and Eve Potts*
> *Avon Books, 1994*

"Coping with Prostate Cancer: A Guide to Living with Prostate
Cancer for You and Your Family"
> *By Robert H. Phillips*
> *Avery Publishing Group, Garden City Park, N.Y., 1994*

"How I Survived Prostate Cancer — and So Can You: A Guide
for Diagnosing and Treating Prostate Cancer"
> *By James Lewis Jr.*
> *Health Education Literary Publishers, Westbury, N.Y., 1994*

"My Prostate and Me: Dealing with Prostate Cancer"
> *By William C. Martin*
> *Cadell & Davies, New York, N.Y., 1994*

"Prostate Cancer: Making Survival Decisions"
> *By Sylvan Meyer and Seymour C. Nash*
> *University of Chicago Press, Chicago, Ill., 1994*

"The Prostate Book: Sound Advice on Symptoms and Treatment"
> *By Stephen N. Rous*
> *Norton, New York, N.Y., 1994*

"BPH (Benign Prostatic Hypertrophy) & Prostate Cancer"
> *By Kurt W. Donsbach*
> *Rockland Corporation, 1993*

"Cancer"
> *By Robert M. McAllister, Sylvia Teich Horowitz and*
> *Raymond V. Gilden*
> *BasicBooks, New York, N.Y., 1993*

"Prostate: Questions You Have — Answers You Need"
    By Sandra Salmans
    People's Medical Society, Allentown, Pa., 1993

"Recovering from Prostate Cancer"
    By Leonard G. Gomella and John J. Fried
    Harper Paperbacks, New York, N.Y., 1993

"The Prostate: Facts and Misconceptions"
    By Hernando Salcedo
    Carol Publishing Group, Secaucus, N.J., 1993

"The Prostate Sourcebook: Everything You Need to Know"
    By Steven Morganstern
    Lowell House, Los Angeles, Calif.; and
    Contemporary Books, Chicago, Ill., 1993

"The Intelligent Guide to Prostate Cancer: All You Need to Know
to Take an Active Part in Your Treatment"
    By Sheldon Larry Goldenberg
    Intelligent Patient Guide, Vancouver, Canada, 1992

"Your Prostate: What Every Man Over 40 Needs to Know —
Now!"
    By Chet Cunningham
    United Research Publishers, Leucadia, Calif., 1991

"Overcoming Bladder Disorders: Compassionate, Authoritative
Medical and Self-help Solutions for Incontinence, Cystitis, Interstitial Cystitis, Prostate Problems and Bladder Cancer"
    By Rebecca Chalker and Kristene E. Whitmore
    Harper & Row, New York, N.Y., 1990

"Dr. Greenberger's What Every Man Should Know About
His Prostate"
    By Monroe E. Greenberger
    Walker, New York, N.Y., 1988

"Prostate Cancer: A Survivor's Guide"
    By Don Kaltenbach and Tim Richards
    Walker, New York, N.Y., 1988

"La Prostata: Sus Enfermedades y Su Tratamiento"
By Gabriel Arvis
Mensajero, Bilbao, 1982

"Recalled By Life"
By Anthony J. Sattilaro and Tom Monte
Houghton Mifflin, Boston, Mass. 1982

"A Private Battle"
By Cornelius Ryan and Katheryn Morgan Ryan
Simon and Schuster, New York, N.Y., 1979

Internet Addresses

Note: these can change periodically and this is only a partial list of what is actually out there, but it is a start.

Prostate

Basic and Clinical Aspects of Prostate Cancer
http://www.secap1.com/prostate/top.html

BPH Diagnosis and Tx
http://www.jr2.ox.ac.uk/Bandolier/band11/b11-3.html

Cancernet
http://www.noah.cuny.edu/cancer/nci/cancernet/201121.html

CaP Cure
http://www.capcure.org

Matthews Foundation for Prostate Cancer Research
mathews@sna.com

Patient Experiences with Prostate Cancer Therapies
http://www2.ari.net/icare/expprost.html

Pca InfoLink
http://www.comed.com.prostate/

Prostate Cancer Research Foundation
http://www.giga.net.au/org/prostate/

Prostate.com
http://www.prostate.com

Prostate Pointers
http://rattler.cameron.edu/prostate/prostate.html

Prostatectomy
http://prostate.urol.jhu.edu/surgery/surg.html

Prostatitis Foundation
http://www.prostate.org/

Impotence

Geddings Osbon Sr. Foundation Impotence Resource Center
http://www.impotence.org/

Successfully Treating Impotence
http://www2.impotent.com/caverject

General/Other Urology

Incontinence on the Internet
http://incontinet.com/

The Oley Foundation
http://www.wizvax.net/oleyfdn
(Support for those who require home parenteral and/or enteral nutrition.)

General Medical/Oncology Resources

American Cancer Society
http://www.cancer.org/acs.html

American Institute for Cancer Research (AICR)
http://www.aicr.org

Cancer Care Inc.
http://www.cancercare.org

CenterWatch: Clinical Trials Listing Service
http://www.centerwatch.com/

Coping magazine
Copingmag@aol.com

CNN-Health
http://cnn.com/HEALTH/index.html

FDA
http://www.fda.gov

International Cancer Alliance (ICA)
http://www.icare.org/icare

National Cancer Institute
http://wwwicic.nci.nih.gov/

OncoLink
http://cancer.med.upenn.edu/

Robert Benjamin Ablin Foundation for Cancer Research
http://www.achiever.com/freempg/mhaythor/

Directories/Searches

CancerNet — National Cancer Institute (NCI)
cancernet@icicc.nci.nih.gov

NIH Guide Database
http://www.med.nyu.edu/keyword.htm

Support Services

Corporate Angel Network (CAN)
http://www.mach2media.com/can
(Provides air transportation to cancer patients seeking treatment far from home.)

Hospice/Legal Issues

Choice in Dying
http://www.choices.org
(Provides counseling regarding preparing and using living wills and medical powers of attorney for health care.)

National Hospice Organization (NHO)
http://www.nho.org

Medical Newsletters and Magazines

Coping magazine
P.O. Box 682268
Franklin, Tenn. 37068-2268
(615) 790-2400
(615) 794-0179 (fax)

Drug Lists
U.S. Food and Drug Administration
(800) 300-7469

Family Urology
300 W. Pratt St., Suite 401
Baltimore, Md. 21201
(410) 727-2908

FDA Consumer Magazine
New Orders, Superintendent of Documents
P.O. Box 3371954
Pittsburgh, Pa. 15250-2233

Oncology News International
c/o APS Medical Marketing Group Inc.
264 Passaic Ave.
Fairfield N.J. 07004-2595

Primary Care and Cancer
17 Prospect St.
Huntington, N.Y. 11743
(516) 424-8900

The ABCs of Prostate Disease
University of Michigan
Section of Urology
1500 E. Medical Center Drive
Ann Arbor, Mich. 48109-6804
(313) 936-6804
(313) 936-9127 (fax)

The Medical Herald
211 E. 43rd St., Suite 1600
New York, N.Y. 10017
(212) 983-3525

The Prostate Cancer Communicator
US TOO International Inc.
930 N. York Road, Suite 50
Hinsdale, Ill. 60521-2993
(630) 323-1002

Urology Times
(218) 723-9477
(218) 723-9437 (fax)

Videos

(Listed by year)

Note: some of these videos can only be seen at your doctor's office, while others can be ordered directly from the production company.

"Prostate Cancer
   Time-Life Video Services, N.Y., N.Y.
   1996

"AMS Sphincter 800 Urinary Prosthesis: Restoring Continence After Prostate Surgery"
   American Medical Systems, Minnetonka, Minn.
   1995

"An Alternative Therapy for Prostate Cancer: Seed Implantation"
   Amersham Healthcare, Arlington Heights., Ill.
   1995

"An Introduction to Proscar (finasteride): Medical Treatment for Symptomatic BPH"
Merck & Co., West Point, Pa.
1995

"Donahue: Prostate Cancer"
Multimedia Entertainment
1995

"Facts on Prostate"
American Cancer Society
1995

"How to Use Your AMS Sphincter 800 Urinary Prosthesis"
American Medical Systems, Minnetonka, Minn.
1995

"Impotence Treatments: Making the Right Choice"
American Medical Systems, Minnetonka, Minn.
1995

"LifeLines: A Guide to Life With Prostate Cancer"
TAP Pharmaceuticals, Deerfield, Ill.
1995

"Lupron Depot 7.5 mg. Your Choice for Treating Prostate Cancer"
TAP Pharmaceuticals, Deerfield, Ill.
1995

"Prostate Cancer: What Everyone Should Know"
TAP Pharmaceuticals, Deerfield, Ill.
1995

"Sex After Prostate Cancer Therapy: Medical Therapy for Erection Problems"
American Cancer Society
1995

"Testicular Self-Examination"
Lange Productions, Hollywood, Calif.
1995

"When Someone You Love Has Prostate Cancer"
Zeneca Pharmaceuticals, Wilmington, Del.
1995

"Straight Talk on Prostate Health Video Recording"
A Vision Entertainment, New York, N.Y.
1994

"Digital Rectal Examination: Setting a New Standard"
Merck & Co., West Point, Pa.
1993

"Enlarged Prostate: Treatment Options"
Lange Productions, Hollywood, Calif.
1993

"Every Man Should Know About His Prostate:
A Disease-awareness Video"
Merck & Co., West Point, Pa.
1993

"Into the Light"
Zeneca Pharmaceuticals, Wilmington, Del.
1993

"Keeping Healthy: Overcoming Prostate Cancer"
Schering Corporation, Kenilworth, N.J.
1993

"Prostate Cancer: Treat to Control"
Lange Productions, Hollywood, Calif.
1993

"Prostate Cancer: Treat to Cure"
Lange Productions, Hollywood, Calif.
1993

"The Prostate Puzzle"
WQED, Pittsburgh, Pa.
1993

"Taking Charge: Managing Advanced Prostate Cancer"
Schering Corporation, Kenilworth, N.J.
1993

"On the Bridge"
Direct Cinema Ltd., Santa Monica, Calif.
1992

"Prostate: Ultrasound and Biopsy"
Lange Productions, Hollywood, Calif.
1992

General Medical References

(Listed by year)

Medical Handbooks

Title: *Fast Facts — Prostate Cancer*
Authors: Kirby, R.S.; Oesterling, J.E.; and Denis, L.J.
Publisher: Health Press, Abingdon, Oxford, U.K.
Date: 1996
Phone: 011-44-0-1235-522147
Fax: 011-44-0-1235-528858

Title: *Fast Facts — Benign Prostatic Hyperplasia*
Authors: Kirby, R.S.; and McConnell, J.D.
Publisher: Health Press, Abingdon, Oxford, U.K.
Date: 1995
Phone: 011-44-0-1235-522147
Fax: 011-44-0-1235-528858

Title: *Patient Pictures – Urological Surgery*
Editor: Kirby, R.S.
Date: 1996
Publisher: Health Press, Abingdon, Oxford, U.K.
Phone: 011-44-0-1235-522147
Fax: 011-44-0-1235-528858

Textbooks

Title: *Devita's Textbook of Medical Oncology*
Editors: Oesterling, J.E.; Fuks, Z.B.; Scher, I; et al
Date: 1997

Publisher: J.B. Lippincott, Hagerstown, Md.
Phone: (800) 777-2295
Fax: (301) 714-2398

Title: *Prostate Cancer*
Authors: Kirby, R.S.; Christmas, T.J.; and Brawer, M.
Date: 1996
Publisher: Mosby
Distributor: Zeneca Pharmaceuticals, Wilmington, Del.

Title: *Smith's General Urology* (fourth edition)
Editors: Tanagho, E.A.; and McAninch, J.W.
Article: "Neoplasms of the prostate gland"
Author: Narayan, P.
Chapter: 22
Pages: 392-433
Date: 1995
Publisher: Appleton & Lange, Stanford, Conn.
Phone: (203) 406-4500

Title: *Campbell's Urology — Volume 2* (sixth edition)
Editors: Walsh, P.C.; Retik, A.B.; Stamey, T.A.;
and Vaughan, E.D. Jr.
Article: "Adenocarcinoma of the prostate"
Authors: Stamey, T.A.; and McNeal, J.E.
Chapter: 29
Pages: 1159-1221
Date: 1992
Publisher: W.B. Saunders and Co., Fort Lauderdale, Fla.
Phone: (800) 545-2522
Fax: (407) 352-3445

Title: *Adult and Pediatric Urology — Volume 2*
Editors: Gillenwater, J.Y.; Grayhack, J.T., Howards, S.S.; and
Duckett, J.W.
Article: "Carcinoma of the prostate"
Authors: Kozlowski, J.M.; and Grayhack, J.T.
Chapter: 34
Pages: 1126-1219
Date: 1987
Publisher: Mosby Yearbook Inc., St. Louis, Mo.
Phone: (800) 426-4545

Support Groups and Other Helpful Organizations

There is a lot of help out there for men with prostate cancer and their loved ones. Below is an alphabetical summary of major national organizations that can put you in touch with support groups and other resources in your area.

Because this list continues to grow, we left some blank spaces for you to add new information.

American Cancer Society (ACS)
1599 Clifton Road N.E.
Atlanta, Ga. 30329-4251
(800) ACS-2345

American Foundation for Urologic Disease (AFUD)
300 W. Pratt St., Suite 401
Baltimore, Md. 21201-2463
(800) 242-2383

American Institute for Cancer Research (AICR)
1759 R St., N.W.
Washington, D.C. 20009
(800) 843-8114 (nutrition hotline)
(202) 328-7744
(202) 328-7226 (fax)
AICR is the only national cancer charity that focuses on the link between diet, nutrition and cancer. AICR also provides information on breast, lung, colon and prostate cancers.

American Urological Association (AUA)
1120 North Charles St.
Baltimore, Md. 21201-5559
(410) 727-1100

Canadian Cancer Society
10 Alcorn Ave., Suite 200
Toronto, Ontario, Canada M4v 3B1
(416) 961-7223

Cancer Care Inc.
1180 Avenue of the Americas
New York, N.Y. 10036
(800) 813-HOPE
(212) 302-2400
(212) 719-0263 (fax)
*Provides free professional counseling, support groups and educational
materials.*

Cancer Research Institute
681 Fifth Ave.
New York, N.Y. 10022
(800) 99-CANCER
(212) 688-7515
(212) 832-9376 (fax)
Supports leading cancer research.

CaP Cure
1250 Fourth St., Suite 360
Santa Monica, Calif. 90401
(310) 458-2873
Fax (301) 458-8074

CHEMOcare
231 North Ave. West
Westfield, N.J. 07090-1428
(800) 55-CHEMO
(908) 233-1103
(908) 233-0228 (fax)
*Provides one-to-one emotional support to patients and families from
trained and certified volunteers who themselves are cancer survivors.*

Choice in Dying
200 Varick St., 10th Floor, Room 1001
New York, N.Y. 10014-4810
(800) 989-WILL
(212) 366-5540
(212) 366-5337 (fax)
Provides counseling regarding preparing and using living wills and medical powers of attorney for health care.

Corporate Angel Network (CAN)
Westchester County Airport Building
White Plains, N.Y. 10604
(914) 328-1313
(914) 328-3938 (fax)
Helps cancer patients in stable condition find free flights, on corporate aircraft, to and from recognized cancer treatment centers.

Families Against Cancer (FACT)
P.O. Box 588
DeWitt, N.Y. 13214
(315) 446-6385
(315) 446-5326 (fax)
FACT is an advocacy group for cancer patients and their loved ones.

Geddings Obson Sr. Foundation
P.O. Box 1593
Augusta, Ga. 30903-1593
(800) 433-4215
Impotence education, services and support.

Impotence Resource Center
P.O. Box 1593
Augusta, Ga. 30903

International Cancer Alliance (ICA)
4853 Cordell Ave., Suite 11
Bethesda, Md. 20814
(800) I-CARE-61
(301) 654-8684 (fax)
Provides a free Cancer Therapy Review, which includes information on specific types of cancer, from diagnosis to treatment.

Make Today Count
c/o Connie Zimmerman
Mid-America Cancer Center
1235 E. Cherokee
Springfield, Mo. 65804-2263
(800) 432-2273
(417) 888-7426 (fax)
A mutual support organization for cancer survivors.

Matthews Foundation for Prostate Cancer Research
817 Commons Drive
Sacramento, Calif. 95825-6655
(800) 234-6284
(916) 927-5218 (fax)
Provides individual answers to prostate-cancer survivors and their families about the disease, its symptoms and treatment.

National Association for Continence (NAFC)
(used to be called Help for Incontinent People)
P.O. Box 8310
Spartanburg, S.C. 29305-8310
(800) BLADDER

National Association of Hospital Hospitality Houses Inc.
4013 W. Jackson St.
Muncie, Ind. 47304
(800) 542-9730
(317) 287-0321 (fax)
Provides information on lodging and support for those receiving medical care away from home.

National Cancer Institute (NCI)
31 Center Drive MSC 2580
Building 31, Room 10A16
Bethesda, Md. 20892-2580

- (800) 4-CANCER (Cancer Information Service)
  A nationwide telephone service for cancer patients and their families, as well as the general public and health care professionals, that answers questions and provides free booklets about cancer.

- (301) 402-5874 (CancerFax)
  Provides treatment summaries, with current data on prognosis, relevant staging and histologic classifications, news and announcements of important cancer-related issues.

National Cancer Survivors Day (NCSD) Foundation
P.O. Box 682285
Franklin, Tenn. 37068-2285
(615) 794-3006
(615) 794-0179 (fax)
NCSD is a nationwide, annual celebration of life for cancer survivors, their loved ones and health care professionals. NCSD is celebrated on the first Sunday in June throughout the United States.

National Coalition for Cancer Survivorship (NCCS)
1010 Wayne Ave., Suite 505
Silver Spring, Md. 20910
(301) 650-8868
(301) 565-9670 (fax)
Raises awareness of cancer survivorship through newsletters and other publications; provides education and advocacy for insurance, employment and legal rights for those with cancer.

National Hospice Organization (NHO)
1901 N. Moore St., Suite 901
Arlington, Va. 22209
(800) 658-8898
(703) 525-5762 (fax)
National nonprofit organization devoted to the promotion of hospice care.

National Institute on Aging Information Center
P.O. Box 8057
Garthersburg, Md. 20898-8057
(800) 222-2225

National Kidney and Urologic Disease Information
Clearinghouse
Box NKUDIC
9000 Rockville Pike
Bethesda, Md. 20892
(301) 654-4415
For information on BPH and its treatment.

National Prostate Cancer Coalition (NPCC)
P.O. Box 354
Baltimore, Md. 21203-0554
(800) 242-2383

The Oley Foundation
214 Hun Memorial
Albany Medical Center A-23
Albany, N.Y. 12208
(800) 776-OLEY
(518) 262-5528 (fax)
Support for those who require home parenteral and/or enteral nutrition.

Patient Advocates for Advanced Cancer Treatments (PAACT)
1143 Parmelee N.W.
Grand Rapids, Mich. 49504
(616) 453-1477
(616) 453-1846 (fax)
*An association for both patients and physicians that provides informa-
tion about diagnostic and therapeutic treatments for prostate cancer.*

Prostate Cancer Support Group Network (PCSN)
300 W. Pratt St., Suite 401
Baltimore, Md. 21201
(800) 828-7866

Prostate Health Council
c/o American Foundation for Urologic Disease Inc. (AFUD)
300 W. Pratt St., Suite 401
Baltimore, Md. 21201-2463
(800) 242-2383

R.A. Bloch Cancer Foundation Inc.
The Cancer Hotline
4410 Main St.
Kansas City, Mo. 64111
(816) 932-8453
(816) 931-7486 (fax)
Provides information, peer counseling, medical second opinions and support groups for those with cancer.

Ronald McDonald House
Ronald McDonald House Charities
1 Kroc Drive
Oak Brook, Ill. 60521
(630) 623-7048
(630) 623-7488 (fax)
Offers lodging for family members of cancer patients being treated away from home.

Sex Information and Education Council of the U.S.
130 W. 42nd St.
New York, N.Y. 10036
(212) 819-9770

The Simon Foundation for Continence
P.O. Box 815
Wilmette, Ill. 60091
(800) 23-SIMON

U.S. Department of Health and Human Services
Public Health Service
Agency for Health Care Policy and Research
Publications Clearinghouse
P.O. Box 8547
Silver Springs, Md. 20907
(800) 358-9295
To get a copy of BPH health guidelines.

U.S. Food and Drug Administration (FDA)
Drug Information Branch
HFD210
5600 Fishers Lane
Rockville, Md. 20857
(301) 827-4573

The Wellness Community
2716 Ocean Park Blvd., Suite 1040
Santa Monica, Calif. 90405-5211
(310) 314-2555
(310) 314-7586 (fax)
Provides free psychosocial support to cancer survivors through 16
facilities nationwide.

US TOO International Inc.
930 North York Road, Suite 50
Hinsdale, Ill. 60521-2993
(800) 808-7866
(630) 323-1002
(630) 323-1003 (fax)
Provides prostate-cancer survivors and their families with emotional
and educational support through an international network of support
groups and a quarterly newsletter.

Notes _____

_____

_____

_____

_____

_____

_____

_____

_____

_____

_____

_____

_____

_____

_____

_____

_____

_____

_____

_____

Prostate
Vocabulary List

Prostate
Vocabulary List

Abdominal-pelvic CT (computed tomography) scan — This is an X-ray scan that images the various organs in the abdomen and pelvis. It is used to determine whether the pelvic lymph nodes have been affected with prostate cancer.

Ablation — "Ablate" means to remove. Cryoablation, for example, is a procedure that uses very cold temperatures to destroy cancerous prostate tissue.

Acid phosphatase — Acid phosphatase, also called prostate-acid phosphatase, or PAP, is a substance produced and released by the prostate; higher levels can indicate prostate cancer. Before the PSA test was developed, a test that measured acid-phosphatase levels was used to detect prostate cancer. While the PSA test is a superior method of cancer detection, some doctors still use the acid-phosphatase test along with PSA to help determine whether cancer has spread beyond the prostate. The normal level for acid phosphatase varies according to the type of assay, or test, used.

Acute bacterial prostatitis — A form of prostatitis (inflammation of the prostate) that is caused by bacteria. Symptoms include painful and difficult urination, pain in the lower back and perineum (area between the scrotum and anus), chills, fever and blood in the urine. This type of prostatitis is usually associated with a urinary tract infection, or UTI.

Adenocarcinoma — "Adeno" means gland and "carcinoma" means cancer. Thus, adenocarcinoma is a type of cancer arising from a gland, such as the prostate. Basically, four types of cancers can grow in the prostate, but more than 95 percent are adenocarcinomas. The other three types of cancers of the prostate are carcinosarcomas, ductal carcinomas and small-cell carcinomas, both of which usually have a poor prognosis.

Adjuvant therapy — A type of therapy that is used in conjunction with the main form of treatment. For example, external-beam radiation therapy can be used as an adjuvant to surgery or as an adjuvant to radioactive-seed implantation (brachytherapy).

Adrenal androgens — The adrenal glands, which sit on top of the kidneys, produce small amounts of male hormones (androgens), including testosterone. While 95 percent of testosterone is produced by the testicles, about 5-10 percent comes from the adrenal glands. The effect of adrenal hormones on prostate cancer is unknown. Some physicians think they can contribute to the spread of prostate cancer while others think that the quantity is not large enough to be of concern. (On the other hand, there is no question that testosterone from the testicles can increase the growth rate of prostate cancer; this is why many patients are treated with antiandrogens and why many patients with advanced prostate disease have their testicles removed.)

Age- and race-specific PSA reference ranges — Several years ago, it was discovered that the normal PSA level tends to rise with age, and a man's racial background can also affect his normal PSA level. This concept has led to the widespread use of "age- and race-specific reference ranges" for determining normal PSA levels. So, although the traditional normal PSA range is between 0-4 ng/ml, the upper limit of normal can be as low as 2.5 ng/ml or as high as 6.5 ng/ml, depending on a man's age and race.

Alpha blockers — Drugs that relax the smooth muscle of the prostate, which can help to relieve the symptoms of benign prostatic hyperplasia, or BPH. Doxazosin (trade name Cardura) and terazosin (trade name Hytrin) are both alpha blockers used to treat BPH. Tamsulosin (made by Yamanouchi) is an alpha blocker that is similar to doxazosin and terazosin in terms of its effectiveness and complications. It may soon gain FDA approval.

Analgesic — A type of medicine or a form of treatment that relieves pain.

Analogue — A chemical or drug synthesized in the lab that is structurally similar to a natural compound that is released in the body. For example, a luteinizing-hormone-releasing hormone (LHRH) analogue looks like the actual LHRH that is found in the human body.

Anastomosis — The place where two different structures are surgically reattached or reconnected after an organ has been removed. For example, during radical prostatectomy (removal of the prostate) the neck of the bladder and the urethra are reconnected, or "anastomosed."

Androgens — These are male hormones, such as testosterone, that are produced by the adrenal glands or the testicles.

Androgen-dependent (hormone-sensitive) cells — These are prostate-cancer cells that depend on hormones to survive, or grow. When their hormonal supply is cut off these cells have trouble functioning. The higher a tumor's percentage of hormone-sensitive cells, the better it will respond to treatment with hormone-blocking therapy.

Androgen-independent (hormone-insensitive) cells — These are prostate-cancer cells that do NOT depend on hormones to survive, or grow. These are more difficult prostate-cancer cells to deal with because antiandrogen therapy does not work on them. The higher a tumor's percentage of hormone-insensitive cells, the less likely it will respond to treatment.

Aneuploid — A term that refers to fast-growing cancer cells. (Also see "flow cytometry.")

Angiogenesis — The formation of new blood vessels. For prostate cancer (or any other cancer) to survive, it needs a blood supply. Therefore, there is increasing research interest in drugs (called antiangiogenesis drugs) that do not allow tumors to grow their own blood vessels.

Antiandrogens — Drugs used in hormonal therapy that do not allow the male hormones testosterone and DHT (dihydrotestosterone) to bind to prostate-cancer cells. Cancer cells that are sensitive to these hormones have more trouble functioning and growing when antiandrogens such as flutamide (Eulexin), bicalutimide (Casodex), or nilutamide (Nilandron) are taken.

Antiandrogen therapy — See "hormonal therapy."

Antibiotic (or antimicrobial) drugs — These are drugs that can kill bacteria.

Anticholinergic drugs — These are medications that can be used to treat urinary incontinence.

Anticoagulant — A substance that does not allow blood to clot. Heparin, Coumadin and aspirin are just three of many drugs that prevent blood from clotting. Such drugs should be avoided before surgery to prevent blood loss.

Artificial sphincter — An implantable device used to treat urinary incontinence (loss of urinary control) that has persisted for a year or more.

Aspirin — See "anticoagulant."

Assay — A test that measures the amount of a certain substance in the body. For example, a PSA test is also called a PSA "assay."

Asymptomatic — This means experiencing no symptoms. When cancer is confined to the prostate, there are usually no symptoms or indications that something is wrong. Therefore, a man should have an annual checkup that includes a digital-rectal exam and a PSA test; this is the only way to detect cancer in its early stages, when the chance of cure is still excellent.

Autodonation of blood — This is when a patient banks his own blood in case he needs a transfusion at a later date. Patients who are planning to undergo radical prostatectomy (surgical removal of the prostate) are often advised to bank their blood in case they experience some blood loss during the operation.

Balloon dilation — This is a treatment for benign prostatic hyperplasia, or BPH, that is no longer frequently used. During balloon dilation, a tiny, deflated balloon is placed through a catheter into the portion of the urethra that runs through the prostate. The balloon is then inflated, which stretches the urethra and allows urine to flow more easily from the bladder. The balloon is then deflated and removed.

Benign — A term that means noncancerous.

Benign prostatic hyperplasia — Also called BPH, this is a noncancerous condition in which the prostate expands outward but at the same time pushes inward and compresses the urethra. BPH can block the flow of urine partially or completely.

Bilateral orchiectomy — The surgical removal of the testicles, also called castration. This procedure stops the body from producing large amounts of testosterone, which in turn slows the growth of prostate cancer. This procedure is only used in men whose cancer has spread beyond the prostate.

Biopsy of the prostate — The sampling of tissue from different areas of the prostate, which is then examined to check for the presence of cancer. In diagnosing prostate cancer, at least six biopsies should be requested, a procedure called a sextant biopsy. A prostate biopsy is usually requested by a doctor if the digital-rectal exam and/or PSA test is abnormal. The biopsy is usually performed with the guidance of transrectal ultrasound, or TRUS.

Bladder — A muscular, pouchlike organ above the prostate that holds and stores urine. One end of the bladder is connected to the ureter, which carries urine from the kidneys; the other is connected to the urethra, which carries urine out of the body through the penis.

Bladder neck —The part of the bladder that opens into the urethra and allows urinary control. Input from the brain can either relax the bladder-neck muscles so that urine can flow out of the bladder and into the urethra (so a person can urinate), or tighten the bladder neck so that urine can remain in the bladder.

Bladder-neck contracture — A complication of surgery in which the bladder neck is scarred. This can cause future urinary problems that may require surgical repair.

Blood-thinning drugs — See "anticoagulant."

Bone scan —This is a procedure in which an X-ray-like picture is taken to see whether prostate cancer has spread to the bones. Also called radionuclide scintigraphy, it involves injecting a chemical, or radioactive tracer, into the bloodstream, which may or may not be attracted to the bones, depending upon the presence of cancer.

BPH — See "benign prostatic hyperplasia."

Brachytherapy — This is also called radioactive-seed implantation, internal radiation therapy or interstitial radiation therapy. A procedure in which small, radioactive seeds (either Iodine 125, Palladium 103, Gold 198, Yitterbium 169 or Iridium 192), each about the size of a grain of rice, are placed within the prostate in and near the cancer. The exact number of seeds placed depends on the size of the man's prostate. These seeds can either be temporarily or permanently implanted. Radioactivity is released in an attempt to destroy the cancer or stop it from growing.

Cancer — A potentially fatal disease, characterized by the abnormal reproduction of cells, in which cell growth is out of control. Cancer can occur anywhere in the body and can spread (metastasize) via the bloodstream or the lymphatic system.

Capsule of the prostate — The outside edge, or wall, of the prostate. If cancer penetrates this wall, it is no longer considered to be localized; it is advanced.

Carcinoma — Cancer that starts on the outside surface of an organ. This outside area is actually called the epithelium.

Carcinosarcoma — A rare tumor of the prostate which is made up of epithelial (carcino) and connective tissue (sarcoma) components. It usually has a poor prognosis.

Cardura — See "alpha blockers."

Casodex — This is an FDA-approved antiandrogen, made by Zeneca, used to treat advanced prostate cancer. Its generic name is bicalutamide.

Castration — See "bilateral orchiectomy."

Catheter — This usually refers to a tube that is inserted through the penis up the urethra and into the bladder. It is used to drain urine from the bladder.

CAT scan — See "computed tomography scan."

Central zone of the prostate — One of the four zones of the prostate. Only 5 percent to 10 percent of prostate cancers begin in this area. The other three zones are called the periurethral zone, the transition zone and the peripheral zone.

Chemotherapeutic drugs — This describes a variety of drugs that can kill cancer cells.

Chronic bacterial prostatitis — A type of prostatitis, or inflammation of the prostate, caused by bacteria. It is associated with chronic urinary tract infections, or UTIs. Symptoms include painful, difficult and frequent urination; and pain in the lower back, penis, perineum (area between the scrotum and anus) and/or pubic area.

Clinical staging of prostate cancer — An estimation of the stage, or severity, of prostate cancer based on the results of the PSA blood test, the digital-rectal exam, the transrectal ultrasound and prostate biopsy.

Clinical trials — Experimental studies that help to evaluate the safety and effectiveness of a new treatment. These studies can be done at major university research centers and at government-run research facilities like the National Institutes of Health, or NIH.

Combined, or double-agent, androgen-deprivation therapy — The use of an antiandrogen with an orchiectomy or an LHRH agonist to interfere with the cancer cells' ability to interact with testosterone. Also called complete hormonal therapy, or CHT, this treatment appears to have an advantage over single-agent androgen deprivation therapy, especially when used for prostate cancer that has just spread locally beyond the prostate (stage C or T3).

Complete hormonal therapy (CHT) — See combined, or double-agent, androgen-deprivation therapy.

Computed tomography scan — Also called a CT, or CAT, scan. This involves a large number of X-rays which, when stacked together, provide a three-dimensional, cross-sectional view of certain structures in the body. A CT scan helps some doctors with prostate-cancer staging. It also can assist in more accurate delivery of external-beam radiation by determining the exact position of the prostate.

Core — A piece of tissue taken during a biopsy procedure. All prostate biopsies should involve taking at least six different cores, also called a sextant biopsy.

Corpus cavernosa and corpus spongiosum — Spongy areas in the penis which, when filled with blood, create an erection. These areas are also the site of self-injections of drugs for the treatment of impotence.

Cryoablation — Also called cryotherapy or cryosurgery. The use of very low temperatures to freeze the prostate and thus kill prostate-cancer cells and/or stop the cancer from growing. The low temperatures are achieved through the use of liquid nitrogen.

Cryosurgery — See "cryoablation."

Cryotherapy — See "cryoablation."

CT scan — See "computed tomography scan."

Cyst- — The prefix for bladder. For example, "cystoscopy" means viewing the bladder with a device.

Cystitis — Inflammation of the bladder, which often causes painful urination. This can be a side effect of radiation therapy or simply the result of a bacterial infection of the bladder.

Cystometry — A procedure in which a tiny catheter is threaded through the urethra into a full bladder to measure the organ's function and pressure.

Cystoscopy — A procedure in which the bladder, prostate and urethra are viewed through a tiny illuminated tube. This allows the doctor to get a better view of these structures.

DES — See "diethylstilbestrol."

DHT — See "dihydrotestosterone."

DIC — See "disseminated intravascular coagulation."

Diethylstilbestrol — A female hormone, commonly called DES, used in the treatment of prostate cancer. It causes the amount of testosterone to decrease, thus starving the cancer of its hormonal fuel.

Differentiation of prostate-cancer cells — Differentiation refers to variations in the appearance of prostate-cancer cells. Subtle differences in the cancer's appearance can help determine how aggressive the cancer is and how it should be treated. There are basically three types of differentiation, or appearance, of prostate-cancer cells:

- **Well-differentiated** — cancer cells that are uniform in shape and close together. They are given a low Gleason score (2, 3 or 4) by the pathologist, and they grow slowly.

- **Moderately differentiated** — cancer cells that have lost some of their uniform shape and are more spread out. They are given a medium Gleason score (5, 6 or 7) by the pathologist, and it is hard to tell whether they will grow fast or slow.

- **Poorly differentiated** — cancer cells that have no real uniform shape and have combined together to form large tumor masses. They are given a high Gleason score (8, 9 or 10) by the pathologist, and they are the most aggressive cancer cells.

Digital-rectal exam — A test, also called a DRE, in which the doctor's gloved and lubricated index finger is inserted into the rectum to feel for any hardness, bumps or enlargement that may indicate cancer or another disorder of the prostate. The exam usually takes five seconds. The DRE should be done along with a PSA test during an annual prostate exam.

Dihydrotestosterone — A stronger form of the male hormone testosterone, also called DHT. Testosterone is changed into DHT in the prostate by an enzyme called five alpha reductase. This enzyme can be blocked by a medication called Proscar (for the treatment of BPH).

Diploid — A term that refers to slow-growing cancer cells. (Also see "flow cytometry.")

Disseminated intravascular coagulation — A blood-clotting disorder, also called DIC, that can occur in some patients with advanced prostate cancer.

Disseminated prostate cancer — Cancer found throughout the prostate or throughout the body. This is the opposite of "focal" prostate cancer, which is found only in one area of the gland.

Diuretics — Drugs that rid the body of excess water through more frequent urination.

Double-agent androgen-deprivation therapy — See "combined, or double-agent, androgen-deprivation therapy."

Double-blind study — This is a type of study in which neither the doctor nor the study participants know who is receiving the active drug being tested; this helps ensure objectivity in evaluating the drug's effectiveness.

Doxazosin — See "alpha blockers."

DRE — See "digital-rectal exam."

Dry ejaculation — A condition, also called retrograde ejaculation, in which semen does not come out of the penis when a man has an orgasm. Instead, the semen flows back into the bladder because the bladder neck is damaged. Dry ejaculation is a complication of transurethral resection and other various prostate procedures.

Ductal carcinoma — A rare tumor of the prostate which begins growing in a prostate duct (ducts are locations of excretions or secretions from a gland, for example the periurethral duct/glands of the prostate). The prognosis of this cancer varies from good to poor.

Edema — Swelling caused by fluid buildup. In the prostate, this can be due to an infection or a type of treatment, such as cryosurgery or radiation therapy.

Ejaculation — The discharging of semen from the penis during orgasm. Semen, also called ejaculate, is made up of sperm cells and fluid produced by a variety of reproductive organs, including the prostate.

Enucleate — This word is usually used in conjunction with prostate-removal surgery, in which the surgeon's fingers are used to remove, or enucleate, prostatic tissue from around the urethra.

Epididymis — The place where sperm is stored after it is made in the testicles. It is where sperm cells begin to mature and acquire the ability to swim, or move.

Epidural anesthesia — The injection of anesthetic into the spine through a thin tube. After the initial dose, additional anesthetic can be given as needed to numb the lower body. The amount of pain relief and the area of numbness can be adjusted with this form of anesthesia, during which the patient remains conscious.

Erectile dysfunction — This is when an erection is not strong enough for sexual intercourse to occur.

Estrogens — female hormones that are also made in small quantities in males, especially as they age. Estrogens are used to block testosterone production in men with advanced prostate cancer. The most commonly used estrogen is DES (diethylstilbestrol), which is taken orally.

Eulexin — An antiandrogen used in the treatment of prostate cancer. Made by Schering, it is also known by the generic name flutamide.

External-beam radiation therapy — A treatment for prostate cancer in which a high dose of radiation is delivered from an outside source (hence the name external) into the prostate to kill the cancer and stop it from growing. This treatment requires the patient to come to the hospital five days a week for four to six weeks. Each treatment session lasts about 15-30 minutes.

Extracapsular prostate tissue — The tissue that immediately surrounds the outside, or capsule, of the prostate. Cancer that has spread to this area and beyond is considered to be advanced disease.

FDA — See "Food and Drug Administration."

Finasteride — This antiandrogen drug, made by Merck, is known by the trade name Proscar. It is an inhibitor of the enzyme five-alpha reductase, which converts testosterone into DHT (dihydrotestosterone, a more powerful form of testosterone). Finasteride also shows promise in preventing prostate cancer and promoting hair growth; its effectiveness in these areas is currently being evaluated.

Five-alpha reductase — An enzyme in the prostate that can convert testosterone into a stronger form of testosterone called DHT, or dihydrotestosterone.

Five-alpha reductase inhibitors — A type of drug that prevents the conversion of testosterone to DHT, or dihydrotestosterone. Proscar (finasteride), made by Merck, is one of these inhibitors and it is used in the treatment of benign prostate enlargement and in the National Prostate Cancer Prevention Trial.

Flow cytometry — This is a process that defines the genetic makeup of cancerous cells as either "diploid" (slow-growing), "aneuploid" or "polyploid" (aggressive, or fast-growing).

Fluoroscopy — This is a moving X-ray image that appears live on a screen as opposed to waiting to see an actual photograph or film. It is used most commonly for viewing the lower urinary tract before and after treatment.

Flutamide — See "Eulexin."

Focal prostate cancer — Cancer found in only one or a few small areas of the prostate.

Foley catheter — A tube that is inserted into the urethra and bladder through the tip of the penis. In addition to draining urine from the bladder, it can be used to irrigate the bladder and prostatic urethra to prevent the formation of blood clots.

Follicle-stimulating hormone — Also called FSH, this hormone stimulates sperm production in the testicles.

Following expectantly — An uncommon name for watchful waiting, the practice of monitoring the course of prostate cancer without immediately pursuing active treatment.

Food and Drug Administration — Also called the FDA, this federal agency approves drugs and treatments for public use. The approval criteria deal with issues of safety and treatment effectiveness.

Frequency — A word used to describe frequent urination.

Frozen sections — During a radical prostatectomy, some of the pelvic lymph nodes are identified, removed and then frozen. They are then cut into thin sections and examined under a microscope to see if they contain cancer.

FSH — See "follicle-stimulating hormone."

Genetic drift — As a cancer grows, it may go from a well-differentiated, slow-growing tumor to a poorly differentiated, aggressive malignancy. This process is called "genetic drift."

Gleason grading system — Named after the pathologist who came up with this system for grading the aggressiveness of a tumor by describing its physical characteristics. On a total scale of 2 to 10, the higher the grade, the more aggressive, or fast-growing, the cancer appears to be.

GnRH — The abbreviation for "gonadotropin-releasing hormone." (Also see "luteinizing-hormone-releasing-hormone.")

Gonadotropin-releasing hormone (GnRH) — See "luteinizing-hormone-releasing-hormone."

Goserelin — The generic name for the antiandrogen drug Zoladex, used to treat advanced prostate cancer.

Growth factors — Molecules in the body that can increase the amount of cell division, or growth. Sometimes they can also stimulate cancer growth. Some of the most powerful chemotherapeutic drugs are believed to work by blocking growth factors that a cancer might need to survive.

Gynecomastia — Enlargement (swelling), tenderness or pain in the breasts of men who undergo certain types of hormonal therapy. This side effect can be treated with radiation if it doesn't resolve on its own.

Heparin — See "anticoagulant."

Hereditary prostate cancer — Prostate cancer can be inherited from either the mother's or father's side of the family. A family has hereditary prostate cancer if:

- three first-degree relatives (a father and at least two brothers) have had prostate cancer at any age;
- two first-degree relatives (a father and one or more brothers) have had prostate cancer before the age of 55; or
- three generations of the family have had a father, grandfather or son with prostate cancer.

Hesitancy — Difficulty in starting urine flow.

High-dose-rate (HDR) prostate brachytherapy (also called temporary iridium template therapy) — This is a temporary radioactive seed implantation procedure. Radioactive iridium seeds are temporarily implanted in the prostate, followed by external beam radiation therapy. The complication rate, time lost, pain and dollar cost with the permanent seed implant procedure is lower than with this procedure, but it seems to have the same results with respect to the local control of cancer.

HIFU — See "high-intensity focused ultrasound."

High-intensity focused ultrasound — This treatment for benign prostatic enlargement, also called HIFU, uses heat from ultrasound energy like a knife to trim excess prostate tissue that may cause urinary problems.

Hormonal therapy — Also called "hormone-deprivation" and "antiandrogen" therapy, this is a treatment for prostate cancer that deprives some cancer cells of the hormones they need to grow. This can be done by removing the testicles or getting a pill or shot that can shut down the production of male hormones.

Hormone-dependent vs. hormone-independent prostate cancer — Hormone-dependent cancer needs hormones from the body to grow and live. If you have prostate cancer it is better to have the hormone-dependent variety, because today's treatments can shut off the hormone production that fuels cancer growth. Hormone-independent cells, on the other hand, can thrive without the presence of hormones — they will continue to grow regardless of whether the hormone supply is cut off. Therefore, some other type of treatment other than hormonal therapy (radiation, surgery or cryosurgery) is needed to try and stop these cells from growing.

Hormone-deprivation therapy — See "hormonal therapy."

Hormones — Types of chemicals that control various bodily functions. Hormones are secreted by various glands and carried through the bloodstream to different organs.

Hot flashes — This is a sudden warm feeling in the face, neck, back or other areas that can last a few seconds, a few minutes or even hours. Some hormonal treatments for prostate cancer cause this effect, which can be reduced or treated with drugs such as Megace (megastrol acetate). This side effect, which occurs in 50 percent of men who undergo hormonal therapy, is more commonly associated with female menopause.

Hot spots — These are images on a bone scan that indicate where prostate cancer has spread to the bones.

Hyperplasia — An increase in the number of cells. This helps to explain why the prostate gets larger in a benign condition called BPH, or benign prostatic hyperplasia.

Hyper-reflexive —This usually refers to a spastic, or overactive, bladder, characterized by urgency (the strong desire to urinate) and urge incontinence (the strong urge that results in urine leakage).

Hyperthermia — Using the heat from microwave radiation to treat benign prostatic enlargement.

Hytrin — See "alpha blockers."

Impotence — Partial or total loss of an erection, which can be caused by a variety of prostate-cancer treatments or by older age. The condition may be temporary or permanent. Regardless of the cause, it can be treated by medication, a vacuum device or the injection of a drug into the penis to increase blood flow to the organ.

Incision — A cut made by a surgeon to get to the structure to be fixed or removed.

Incontinence — The partial or total loss of urinary control that can occur from a variety of prostate-cancer treatments or from advanced age. Incontinence can be treated with an artificial sphincter or by collagen injections.

Infectious prostatitis — Also called chronic or acute bacterial prostatitis, a type of inflammation of the prostate.

Internal radiation therapy — See "brachytherapy."

Interstitial radiation therapy — See "brachytherapy."

Intravenous — The delivery of fluids and nutritional supplements into the body through a vein, usually in the arm, also called an "IV."

Invasive — A term used to describe any test or procedure that requires an incision.

Investigational treatment —A treatment or device that has NOT been approved by the FDA. This does not mean it is ineffective or unsafe, just that there has not been enough data collected to make a solid decision regarding its approval.

IV — See "intravenous."

Kegel exercises — Exercises that may help strengthen the muscles involved in urination. These exercises are done by stopping and starting the flow of urine and by squeezing and tightening the buttocks while standing to urinate.

Kidneys — These organs filter toxins from the blood, which are then excreted in the urine. The kidneys are connected to the ureters, which lead to the bladder. Urine then travels from the bladder into the urethra, the tube that carries urine from the penis.

Laparoscopic pelvic lymphadenectomy — This procedure involves making a small abdominal incision through which a viewing tube is placed. It allows the doctor to look at the lymph nodes near the prostate and to biopsy them with long, thin surgical instruments. This procedure can help with the staging of prostate cancer. It is also used to observe the inside of the abdomen.

Lateral-lobe enlargement — A type of benign prostatic hyperplasia, or enlargement, in which prostate tissue squeezes the sides of the urethra and thus can cause urinary problems.

Leuprolide — The generic name for the prostate-cancer drug Lupron, which shuts of the production of testosterone.

Luteinizing hormone (LH) — A brain hormone that stimulates testosterone production in the testicles.

Luteinizing-hormone-releasing-hormone (LHRH) — Also known as GnRH, or gonadotropin-releasing hormone. This is a hormone made in the brain that stimulates the release of LH (luteinizing hormone), which in turn stimulates testosterone production.

LHRH agonist — A synthetic (man-made) hormone that is structurally similar to LHRH (luteinizing-hormone-releasing-hormone). When administered as a drug, it shuts down the production of LH (luteinizing hormone), which in turn halts testosterone production. This type of drug is used to treat prostate cancer by depriving the cancer of its "fuel," testosterone.

Libido — Another word for sex drive. A person with a strong sex drive is said to have a strong libido.

Localized prostate cancer — Cancer that is confined to the prostate.

Lupron — See "leuprolide."

Lymphadenectomy — The removal of lymph nodes near the prostate to help with the staging process. Also called lymph-node dissection. Determining whether the lymph nodes are positive, or cancerous, helps define a patient's long-term outcome and treatment options.

Lymph-node dissection — See "lymphadenectomy."

Lymph nodes — Lymph nodes are bean-shaped pockets of lymphocytes (immune-system B cells) held together by fibrous tissue. Lymph nodes are found throughout the body, especially in the neck, underarm and pelvis. Being part of the immune system, lymph nodes help fight disease. If cancer is found in the lymph nodes this is a good indication that the cancer escaped a nearby structure. For example, if someone has prostate cancer and malignant cells are also found in the pelvic lymph nodes, it means that the cancer has gone beyond the prostate. This information has a major impact on the patient's treatment options.

Magnetic resonance imaging — An imaging procedure, also called MRI, that uses magnetism and radio waves rather than X-rays to produce a picture of the inside of the body. An MRI may be used to see whether there is cancer in the prostate and if it has spread to neighboring structures. The procedure involves lying inside an enclosed space for about 45 minutes, so it can be difficult for those who are claustrophobic, or do not like to be in confined spaces.

Malignant — A term that means cancerous.

Margin of the prostate — This refers to the outside surface of the prostate gland. If cancer has invaded the margin it is called "margin positive" and if it has not invaded this area it is called "margin negative."

Maximal androgen blockade — See "combined androgen deprivation therapy."

Metastasis (the plural form is metastases) — The spread of cancer beyond its primary location to other sites in the body such as the bones, lungs, bloodstream or other nearby structures.

Middle-lobe enlargement — This is a form of benign prostatic hyperplasia, or BPH, in which part of the prostate grows up into the bladder. This tissue can partially or totally block the drainage of urine from the bladder into the urethra.

Minilap — See "mini-laparotomy."

Mini-laparotomy — In this procedure, also called a "minilap" or a "staging pelvic lymphadenectomy," a small incision is made, through which the pelvic lymph nodes are examined. If they are not cancerous, the incision is enlarged and the prostate is surgically removed. If the nodes are found to have cancer, the incision is closed and other treatment options are considered.

Moderately differentiated — See "differentiation of prostate-cancer cells."

Monotherapy – "See single agent androgen deprivation therapy."

MRI — See "magnetic resonance imaging."

National Cancer Institute — This government organization, also called the NCI, is an arm of the National Institutes of Health, or NIH, located in Bethesda, Md. The NCI organizes and funds many clinical research trials and helps establish guidelines for cancer treatment and research in the United States.

NCI — See "National Cancer Institute."

Neoadjuvant hormonal therapy — This is the use of hormonal therapy to shrink or contain the prostate cancer prior to radical prostatectomy (surgical removal of the prostate) or radiation therapy.

Nerve-sparing radical prostatectomy — An operation to remove the prostate that allows at least one of the two nerve bundles near the gland to be saved. Sparing these nerves greatly increases a man's chance of retaining normal sexual function.

Neurovascular bundles — Two bundles of nerves and blood vessels, one located on each side of the prostate, that help a man achieve an erection. Removal of or injury to both nerve bundles results in impotence. Sparing at least one of these bundles in most cases allows a man to keep having normal erections.

Ng/ml — The abbreviation for "nanograms per milliliter." A nanogram is one-billionth of a gram, and a milliliter is one-thousandth of a liter. Whenever a man gets a PSA test, the result is reported in nanograms per milliliter, or ng/ml. For example, a PSA test result of 3 actually means 3 ng/ml. The larger the number, the higher the level of PSA in the bloodstream.

NIH — See "National Cancer Institute."

Nilandron — An antiandrogen used in the treatment of prostate cancer. Made by Hoechst Marion Roussel, it is also known by the generic name nilutamide.

Nocturia — Waking up many times in the night to urinate, a common symptom of benign prostatic hyperplasia, or BPH.

Nonbacterial prostatitis — Inflammation of the prostate, the cause of which is unknown. Symptoms include painful, difficult urination and pain in the penis, scrotum, perineum, lower back and general pubic area.

Noninvasive — A medical test or procedure in which no incision is necessary. For example, an ultrasound examination is noninvasive.

Nuclear medicine — This is the department in the hospital where bone scans are usually performed. Bone scans help the doctor to determine whether a man's prostate cancer has spread into the skeleton.

Oncologist — A doctor who treats cancer patients. An oncologist is also qualified to do a prostate checkup. Oncologists can be specialized in a specific type of cancer treatment. For example, a radiation oncologist specializes in the treatment of cancer using radiation.

Orchiectomy — See "bilateral orchiectomy."

Organ-confined — This refers to cancer that is still entirely located within the organ or gland in which it started.

Orgasm — Sexual climax, characterized by ejaculation in men.

Overflow incontinence — Urine leakage caused by a full bladder.

Palliative treatment — This is any treatment that reduces the symptoms of cancer but does not cure it. For example, palliative radiation therapy (also called spot radiation) helps to reduce bone pain associated with advanced prostate cancer but does not cure the cancer.

PAP — See "acid phosphatase."

Pathologist — A doctor who examines the tissues and cells of the body under a microscope to determine what type of disease is present. A pathologist will assign a Gleason score to the prostate cancer and also help stage the disease. A pathologist specializing in urological problems such as prostate cancer is called a uro-pathologist.

Pathological staging of prostate cancer — The evaluation of the prostate tissue removed during surgery to determine how far the cancer has spread.

Pelvic area — This is the area of the body below the waist, including the genital region.

Penile — This refers to anything related to the penis. For example, penile implants help to make the penis erect.

Penile implants — Mechanical, inflatable and bendable devices that, once surgically inserted into the penis, help with erectile dysfunction and impotence.

Perineum — The area between the scrotum (the sac that holds the testicles) and anus.

Peripheral zone of the prostate — The largest part of the prostate, where about 70 percent of all prostate cancers begin to grow. This is also the only area of the gland that can be felt during a digital-rectal exam.

Periprostatic tissue — This is the tissue just outside the prostate. If cancer has spread to the periprostatic tissue, then it is no longer localized, or confined.

Periurethral zone of the prostate — The smallest zone of the prostate, which surrounds the urethra. Cancer rarely begins growing in this area.

Placebo — This is a pill or other substance that contains no real medicine. In some studies, placebos are given to one group of unsuspecting patients while another group unknowingly receives a real drug. The reactions of the two groups are then compared to test the effectiveness of the real medication.

Placebo effect — This is a commonly observed phenomenon in which people receiving a placebo actually have some improvement in their symptoms, even though the pill or substance they have been taking contains no real medicine.

Polyploid — An extra set of chromosomes, which could indicate an abnormal or cancerous cell. Recent blood tests (flow cytometry, static image analysis) can detect polyploid cells in the bloodstream, which could indicate that a cancer has grown beyond the prostate.

Poorly differentiated — See "differentiation of prostate-cancer cells."

Proctitis — Inflammation of the rectum. This can be a side effect of radiation therapy, but it usually lasts for a short time. Symptoms include rectal bleeding, pain and diarrhea.

Prognosis — This is an estimation of how good or bad the patient will do in the future based on all of the available medical information, including the treatment the person is currently undergoing.

Proscar — See "finasteride."

Prostate — A muscular, walnut-shaped gland located below the bladder and above the rectum. The prostate produces about a third of the fluid that makes up semen. This fluid nourishes the sperm and helps them survive inside the woman's body so pregnancy has a better chance of occurring.

Prostate-acid phosphatase — See "acid phosphatase."

Prostate-specific antigen — Also called PSA, this is a product made by the prostate that leaks into the blood. High levels of PSA in the circulation can indicate prostate cancer or benign enlargement of the gland. An annual prostate checkup should include both a PSA blood test and a digital-rectal exam.

Prostatectomy — This is a procedure that involves either partial or complete removal of the prostate.

Prostatic urethra — The portion of the urethra that goes through the prostate.

Prostatism — This refers to the symptoms associated with benign prostatic hyperplasia, such as a weak urine stream and difficulty urinating.

Prostatitis — An inflammation of the prostate. There are four types of prostatitis: acute bacterial, chronic bacterial, nonbacterial and prostatodynia.

Prostatodynia — This is a type of prostatitis, or inflammation of the prostate. This actually means "painful prostate." The symptoms of prostatodynia include painful, difficult and frequent urination.

Prosthesis — This is a replacement for a part of the body that is not completely functioning or a part of the body that is missing. For example, many types of penile prostheses are used today to help men with erectile dysfunction.

Prostrate — Probably the most common misspelling of the word "prostate."

PSA — See "prostate-specific antigen."

PSA density — This is a formula used to determine a person's chances of having prostate cancer and thus the need for a biopsy. It involves dividing the PSA value (in ng/ml) by the volume, or size, of the prostate (based on transrectal ultrasound).

PSA velocity — The change in PSA level over time. The currently accepted normal annual PSA increase is 0.75 ng/ml. PSA velocity is particularly useful in monitoring two types of patients: those whose PSA level is increasing rapidly but is still within the normal range, and those with a suspiciously high PSA level who have normal biopsy results.

Radiation therapy — This is a general term to describe radiation treatment. However, radiation treatment can come from an outside source (external-beam radiation therapy) or it can come from an internal source (radioactive seed implants).

Radical prostatectomy — Surgical removal of the prostate. There are two types of radical prostatectomy: "retropubic," in which an incision is made in the abdomen; and "perineal," in which an incision is made between the scrotum and anus.

Radioactive-seed implantation — See "brachytherapy."

Radioactive scintigraphy — See "bone scan."

Radiotherapy — Treatment with radiation.

Rectal exam — See "digital-rectal exam."

Rectum — The lower part of the small intestine that ends at the anus.

Recurrence —When cancer returns after initial treatment.

Refractory — This refers to cancer that no longer responds to treatment.

Remission — When cancer successfully responds to treatment. Remission can be temporary or permanent.

Retrograde ejaculation — See "dry ejaculation."

Risk factor — Something that increases a person's chances of getting a disease, such as cancer. For example, a high-fat and low-fiber diet may increase an individual's chance of getting prostate cancer.

Salvage therapy — This is a term used to describe a situation where the first line of treatment did not work and now another type of treatment is being tried. For example, if a radical prostatectomy is not successful, external-beam radiation treatment may then be used.

Sandwich approach — When a patient is given a week off about halfway through external-beam radiation therapy. This gives the bowel and bladder a chance to recover from the shock of treatment.

Scrotum — The pouch of skin that holds the testicles.

Semen — Part of the ejaculate (produced during male orgasm) that contains fluid and sperm. The sperm comes from the testicles and the fluid comes mostly from the prostate and the seminal vesicles.

Seminal vesicle — A reproductive organ that is located close to the urethra and contributes about two-thirds of the fluid for semen. It is also a neighbor to the prostate and a place where prostate cancer may spread.

Sextant biopsy — See "biopsy of the prostate."

Single-agent androgen-deprivation therapy — when a orchiectomy or LHRH agonist is used to interfere with the cancer cells' ability to interact with testosterone. This appears to be almost or just as effective as combined hormonal therapy for advanced prostate cancer.

Sphincter — Muscle tissue that helps to open or close a body opening. For example, when the bladder sphincter opens, urine flows down into the urethra; when it closes, the bladder fills with urine.

Spot radiation — This is external-beam radiation treatment for bone pain associated with advanced prostate cancer. Radiation targeted to painful areas of bone does not stop the cancer from growing, but it can help ease some of the pain.

Staging — A process involving a series of tests to determine how far cancer has spread. In prostate cancer, stage T1 or T2 (also called A or B) means the cancer has not spread beyond the prostate. Stage T3 and T4 (also called C or D) means the cancer has spread beyond the prostate.

Staging pelvic lymphadenectomy — See "mini-laparotomy."

Stress incontinence — This is a type of urinary incontinence caused by normal activities such as walking, lifting or playing tennis.

Strontium — This is an injectable radioactive substance that helps control the pain of prostate cancer that has spread to the bones.

Suramin — An experimental medicine used for the treatment of advanced prostate cancer.

Surgical margins — This refers to the outer margins, or edges, of a prostate gland that has been surgically removed. A pathologist will examine these edges to see if they are free of cancer. If they are cancer-free, then there is a good chance the cancer did not go beyond the prostate and all of it was removed. If the margins contain cancer, chances are the disease has spread beyond the prostate.

Sutures — These are stitches used to close an incision at the conclusion of an operation.

Symptomatic — This means a person is feeling the effects of a disease. For example, one of the many possible effects, or symptoms, of advanced prostate cancer is lower-back pain.

Tamsulosin — See "alpha blockers."

Terazosin — See "alpha blockers."

Temporary iridium template therapy — See high-dose-rate (HDR) brachytherapy.

Testicles (testes) — Part of the male genitals, the testes are located below the penis, inside the scrotum. They produce sperm and most of the body's testosterone.

Testosterone — Testosterone is the hormone responsible for masculine characteristics such as facial and body hair, muscle mass and a deep voice. While the majority of testosterone is made in the testicles, a small portion is produced by the adrenal glands. Testosterone fuels the growth of certain types of prostate-cancer cells, called hormone-dependent cells.

Transition zone of the prostate — The innermost part of the prostate that surrounds the urethra as it leaves the bladder. This is where benign prostatic hyperplasia occurs, as well as a small percentage (15 percent to 20 percent) of prostate cancers.

Transrectal — This refers to any procedure that is done through the rectum, such as ultrasound imaging and biopsy of the prostate.

Three-dimensional treatment planning and conformal therapy — A type of external-beam radiation therapy that uses computerized images from a CT scan to help precisely conform the radiation beam to the shape of the tumor. This allows the delivery of the most powerful dose of radiation to the prostate while minimizing the risk of damage to surrounding structures.

Total androgen blockade — See "combined androgen-deprivation therapy."

Transrectal ultrasound, or TRUS — This diagnostic procedure uses sound waves to obtain a picture of the prostate by placing an ultrasound probe into the rectum.

Transrectal ultrasound (TRUS)-guided biopsy of the prostate — A prostate biopsy is performed under the guidance of transrectal ultrasound, in which sound waves from a rectal ultrasound probe act as a navigator to let the doctor accurately locate the prostate for tissue sampling. A tiny needle is then inserted alongside the probe to remove a small sample of prostate tissue. Usually a minimum of six individual biopsies are taken from different areas of the prostate.

Transurethral resection of the prostate — Also called TURP, this is a treatment for benign prostatic hyperplasia in which fragments of the enlarged prostate are removed to help improve urine flow. TURP is performed through a catheter inserted into the penis, so there is no incision involved.

Treatment-planning CT scan of the prostate — This involves using a CT scan to get a better understanding of the exact position of the prostate. This helps plan the most effective way to deliver radiation during treatment.

Tumor — An abnormal growth that can be malignant (cancerous) or benign (noncancerous).

TURP — See "transurethral resection of the prostate."

Urethra — The channel through which urine and semen are carried from the body through the tip of the penis. While sperm and urine pass through the urethra, they never travel together.

Urethral sphincter — The muscle located just below the penis which, along with the bladder neck, is responsible for urinary control.

Urethral stricture — The scarring and narrowing of the urethra, often a complication of surgical treatment for prostate disease.

Urgency — The feeling of immediately having to urinate.

Urinary incontinence — The loss of some or all urinary control, resulting in the leakage of urine from the bladder.

Urinary retention — When the bladder cannot empty and remains completely or partially full.

Urologist — A surgeon who specializes in diseases and problems associated with the kidneys, bladder and prostate. This kind of doctor is also qualified to do a prostate exam.

Vas deferens — The vas deferens is a tube that carries sperm into the urethra during orgasm.

Vacuum-erection device — A device used by men who can no longer achieve an erection naturally. It consists of a tube that is placed over the penis, through which a vacuum is created that draws blood into the organ. The tube is then removed and a ring is placed at the base of the penis to keep the erection from subsiding. The ring can be left in place for up to 30 minutes.

Watchful waiting — When a man diagnosed with prostate cancer decides to carefully monitor the progress of his cancer rather than opting for immediate treatment. This is an active process that involves the patient and the doctor.

Well-differentiated prostate cancer — See "differentiation of prostate-cancer cells."

Zoladex — See "goserelin."

Coming soon from the authors of
The ABCs of Prostate Cancer:

The ABCs of Prostate Disease

The first medical journal written for a nonmedical audience

featuring:

- easy-to-read information on the latest treatment and research regarding prostate cancer, benign prostatic hyperplasia (BPH), prostatitis and other urologic diseases
- guest articles and editorials by prostate-disease experts
- patient-written stories
- articles by — and for — the wives and partners of men with prostate disease
- tips on coping with the emotional and physical side effects of treatment
- support group information
- conference summaries
- and much, much more!

Thank you for supporting prostate-cancer research!

Profits from this book are dedicated to helping find a cure for prostate cancer. To thank you for your support, we'd like to send you a complimentary copy of the first issue of our new journal, *The ABCs of Prostate Disease*, with no further obligation.

To receive your complimentary issue and information on how to become a charter subscriber, please detach and send in the form below:

- -

❏ Yes, I'd like to receive a free issue of *The ABCs of Prostate Disease* and subscription information with NO OBLIGATION TO BUY.

Name: _____

Address: _____

_____

Daytime phone: _____

Fax: _____

University of Michigan Medical Center
ABCs of Prostate Disease
Section of Urology
1500 E. Medical Center Drive
Ann Arbor, Mich. 48109-0330